The Cultural Politics of the Paralympic Movement

Do the Paralympic Games empower the disability sport community?

Like many other contemporary sporting institutions, the Paralympic Games have made the transition from pastime to spectacle, and the profile of athletes with disabilities has been increased as a result. This book reviews the current status of the Paralympics and challenges the mainstream assumption that the Games are a vehicle for empowerment of the disabled community.

Using ethnographic methods unique in this area of study, P. David Howe has undertaken an innovative and critical examination of the social, political and economic processes shaping the Paralympic Movement. In *The Cultural Politics of the Paralympic Movement* he presents his findings and offers a new insight into the relationship between sport, the body and the culture of disability. In doing so he has produced the most comprehensive and radical text about high-performance sport for the disabled yet published.

P. David Howe is Lecturer in the Sociology of Sport at Loughborough University. He is also a four-time Paralympian and former Athlete's Representative to the International Paralympic Committee.

Routledge Critical Studies in Sport
Series Editors
Jennifer Hargreaves and Ian McDonald
University of Brighton

The Routledge Critical Studies in Sport series aims to lead the way in developing the multi-disciplinary field of Sport Studies by producing books that are interrogative, interventionist and innovative. By providing theoretically sophisticated and empirically grounded texts, the series will make sense of the changes and challenges facing sport globally. The series aspires to maintain the commitment and promise of the critical paradigm by contributing to a more inclusive and less exploitative culture of sport.

Also available in this series:

The Cultural Politics of the Paralympic Movement

Through an anthropological lens

P. David Howe

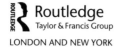 Routledge
Taylor & Francis Group

LONDON AND NEW YORK

First published 2008
by Routledge
2 Park Square, Milton Park, Abingdon, Oxon OX14 4RN

Simultaneously published in the USA and Canada
by Routledge
270 Madison Ave, New York, NY 10016

Routledge is an imprint of the Taylor & Francis Group, an informa business

© 2008 P. David Howe

Typeset in Goudy by Wearset Ltd, Boldon, Tyne and Wear
Printed and bound in Great Britain by TJ International Ltd, Padstow,
Cornwall

British Library Cataloguing in Publication Data
A catalogue record for this book is available from the British Library

Library of Congress Cataloging in Publication Data
A catalog record for this book has been requested

ISBN10: 0-415-28886-X (hbk)
ISBN10: 0-415-28887-8 (pbk)
ISBN10: 0-203-50609-X (ebk)

ISBN13: 978-0-415-28886-6 (hbk)
ISBN13: 978-0-415-28887-3 (pbk)
ISBN13: 978-0-203-50609-7 (ebk)

For TSP, who knew that running would be my salvation.

Contents

Illustrations

Figures

Table

Series editors' foreword

Perhaps more than any other book in the Routledge Critical Studies in Sport Series, this really is the product of a lifetime's personal, sporting and political engagement. It is the culmination of three decades of immersion in the culture of disability sport by P. David Howe, as an athlete, activist and anthropologist. As a result of being an authentic insider to the field, David has produced a highly original text about an increasingly significant movement in sport: the Paralympic Movement.

The Paralympic Movement has enjoyed a good press in recent years. After years of mild ridicule followed by active marginalisation within the mainstream sporting world, the Paralympic Games now receives the kind of attention and support befitting an international mega-sporting event. 'Building on ability' has been the politicised raison d'être for disability sport for more than twenty years now, and as a result disabled athletes have increased in numbers and skilfulness at the grass-roots and are now a recognised part of elite sport. The Paralympic Games has secured a place on the sporting calendar, albeit as a kind of post-script to the main Olympic story; and disabled Olympians are finally receiving recognition for their sporting ability, albeit mainly in certain techno-fashionable events.

How do we make sense of this 'progress'? Has it come at a cost? What has been the impact of the rise of the Paralympic Movement on the culture of disability sport? How are the Paralympic Games positioned within the Olympic Movement? Can disability sport ever receive comparable treatment and respect on a par with able-bodied sport? As part life-history, part insider account and part critique, Howe offers a unique perspective that gets to grip with the complexities and contradictions of disability sport and the Paralympic Movement in the twenty-first century.

The Cultural Politics of the Paralympic Movement fits neatly into the philosophy of the Routledge Critical Studies in Sport Series. When discussing ideas with potential authors, we always emphasise the importance of critique. Our notion of critique can be encapsulated by what we rather playfully refer to as the three 'I's:

Interrogative: the critique challenges common-sense ideas and exposes relations of power in the world of sport;

Interventionist: the critique highlights the relationship between theory and practice and provides arguments and analyses of topical and polemical issues;
Innovative: the critique seeks to develop new areas of research, and stimulate new ways of thinking about and studying sport.

Underpinning our critique is a set of politics, values and beliefs about the role of sport in society. Without being programmatic or didactic, we are committed to developing the multi-disciplinary field of Sport Studies for university students and to maintaining a critical approach to the excessively commercialised, damaging and exploitative culture of top-level competitive sport. *The Cultural Politics of the Paralympic Movement* is a most valuable and necessary addition to the series, integral both to the politics of exclusion and to the critique of the increasing commodification of sport for all people at all levels.

Jennifer Hargreaves and Ian McDonald
Co-editors, Routledge Critical Studies in Sport

Acknowledgements

Those around me will know that this book has been a long time coming. Thank you all for your support. The idea for this monograph first came to me more than twenty years ago, and as a result there was a tremendous amount of data to sift in order to develop an ethnographic account that fully reflects my interpretation.

Thank you to Samantha Grant at Routledge for her patience in waiting for this monograph. I am hopeful it was worth the wait. I am also grateful to Jennifer Hargreaves and Ian McDonald, the series editors, for suggesting this volume. To colleagues in the field of sport studies who have help shape my ideas, particularly Alan Bairner, Jayne Caudwell, Karen DePauw, Dominic Malcolm, Andy Parker and Andy Pitchford, thank you. I have enjoyed our intellectual games.

Many people within the Paralympic Movement have contributed both directly and indirectly to the final project. Thanks in particular to Marie Dannhaeuser, Patrick Jarvis, Blair Miller, Brian Scobie and Eli Wolff, who made me realise I had a story to tell. I am grateful to those who helped me in all forms of training throughout this project. For my training in the field of anthropology, thanks go to Ron Vastokas, Gavin Smith and Murray Last. They have all taught me how to be a better ethnographer. Thanks also to Alan Klein and Gary Armstrong, who have shown me through word and deed that the anthropology of sport is a worthwhile pursuit, and to TSP, Scott Ogilvie, Mike Sherar and Steve Pritchard for training my imperfect mortal engine.

Finally, a big thank you to my family, without whose support I would not have been encouraged to lead a 'normal' life. Thanks also to my partner Carol, who took on the role as my personal editor with gusto. The monograph has no doubt been improved as a result.

Abbreviations

CASD	IPC Commission for Athletes with a Severe Disability
CIAD	Commission for the Inclusion of Athletes with a Disability
CP-ISRA	Cerebral Palsy International Sports and Recreation Association
EAD	Elite Athletes with a Disability
EPC	European Paralympic Committee
IBC	International Boccia Commission
IBSA	International Blind Sports Association
ICC	International Coordinating Committee of the World Sports Organisations
ICF	International Classification of Functioning, Disability, and Health
INAS-FID	International Association of Sport for Persons with an Intellectual Disability
INAS-FMH	International Sports Federation for Persons with Mental Handicap
IOC	International Olympic Committee
IPC	International Paralympic Committee
IPCAC	International Paralympic Committee Athletics Committee
ISMWSF	International Stoke Mandeville Wheelchair Sports Federation
ISOD	International Sports Organisation for the Disabled
IWAS	International Wheelchair and Amputee Sport Association

1 Athlete as anthropologist, anthropologist as athlete

> To be disabled is tragic enough but also to be excluded totally from the pleasures of physical recreation and sport is to be doubly unfortunate.
>
> (Bannister 1977: 64)

When the quotation above was penned just over three decades ago, the attitude expressed would have been seen by those in the medical fraternity as somewhat enlightened. This would not be the case today, particularly if you, the reader, have experience of the contemporary Paralympic Movement. In the public consciousness it would be seen as politically inappropriate to refer to an impairment as tragic. Today an impairment may offer resistance to achievement in one's chosen field of endeavour, but we all face certain obstacles on the way to our goals. Recently there has been a push to establish rights for the disabled communitas[1] globally. In 2006 the United Nations established a Treaty on Rights for the Disabled that included issues regarding access to sport and leisure provision (article 30), which it is hoped will go some way to addressing issues of access to sporting and leisure provision for all.

Over the past twenty years there has been massive change in elite sport for the disabled. It has been widely accepted within disability-studies circles that a person-first approach should be adopted when addressing athletes with a disability (see, for example, Oliver 1990; Barnes and Mercer 2003). In this monograph I have stuck to this convention except when referring to sport as an institution. When the phrase 'sport for the disabled' is used instead of 'disability sport' it is because, through my research, it has become clear that sporting provision for the disabled is part of what might be labelled a 'disability industry' (Albrecht and Bury 2001). Therefore, because Paralympic sport is run largely by the 'able', the phrase 'sport for the disabled' seems appropriate. While some familiar with this field of study may see my use of the term 'sport for the disabled' as outdated, to explore the cultural politics of the Paralympic Games properly it is vital that researchers and readers alike are reminded that social oppression does not evaporate with a change in lexicon.

Disabled activists and theorists (Oliver 1990, 1996; Morris 1991, 1996) also make the distinction between impairment, an acquired or born trait, and disability, the wider impact of the social context of these impairments. Impairment is a functional trait, or in lay terms what is 'wrong with a person', which often has consequences regarding whether the person's body is seen as 'normal'. It has been suggested that 'Impairment does not necessarily create dependency and a poor quality of life; rather it is lack of control over the physical help needed which takes away people's independence' (Morris 1996: 10). By extension it appears that sport for the impaired might be a more appropriate term than 'sport for the disabled', yet the former lacks the overt political connotation that is culturally relevant to the current study.

Sport for the disabled is a practice that is in need of close examination. The cultural politics of the relationships between the concepts of disability and impairment can be examined through a detailed ethnographic investigation. The monograph you are reading is one of the products of a diachronic study of the cultural politics of the Paralympic Movement. This research will illuminate the structural importance of sport for the disabled, but also highlight how the impaired sporting body should be central to any such study of sport for the disabled.

In the past sixty years sport for the disabled has gone from being a platform for the rehabilitation of war-wounded to the point where the Paralympic Games is the most recognised sporting festival for people with impairments. Paralympic sport has gone from providing athletes with the opportunity of participation to adopting a high-performance model of sporting practice that attracts a large amount of media attention. This volume is designed to illuminate this transformation ethnographically in order to give those unfamiliar with the high-performance component of sport for the disabled an insight into this distinctive cultural milieu. Because of the nature of the methods used in ethnographies (see Appendix 1) this monograph focuses upon track and field athletics, as this is the sporting practice in which I have been and continue to be involved. Athletics is arguably the flagship sport of the Paralympic Movement, and so those with interests in other sports may be able to see similarities in analysis and interpretation. The focus on athletics should not be seen as a statement of the lack of importance of other sports as fields of study, but rather that my limited capital as an athlete is tied to the sport of athletics and hence it is the focus of this monograph.

There are numerous reasons why academics write books. Some engage in the process to advance themselves professionally, others because they believe in providing a 'public' outlet for their research, and some simply because they think that they have something to contribute to wider intellectual debate. This book is the product of all of these reasons and is, as far as I could manage, written in the form that it is simply because an ethnographic monograph has a validity above all other forms of writing within the discipline of social anthropology. Yet before the monograph starts in earnest, I want to address the issue of my positioning in the 'field' of the Paralympic Movement, starting with early memories and progressing to the point where I began to realise that I was an ethnographer ideally positioned to tell the story that will unfold throughout this work.

Into the field

As a former Paralympian who represented Canada in each summer Paralympic Games from 1988 until 2000 in the sport of track and field athletics, and then worked as a member of the media for a British magazine *Run, Throw and Jump*[2] during the 2004 Games, some readers might expect this account to be autobiographical. It is not. In recent years there have been calls for ethnography to embrace autobiography (Davies 1997). The development of autoethnography has, to a degree, become a useful tool in the continued exploration of the social significance of sport (see Sparkes 2002), yet this book is not designed to be part of the genre, preferring to engage in an ethnographic account that makes explicit my presence in the field while not situating myself at its centre (see Coffey 1999). In the field of anthropology the way in which a monograph is constructed changes as styles ebb and flow, so no doubt there will be those who read this text and believe it could have better served the academic communitas and, to a lesser extent, the public if it had been written in another format. The difficulty is that by trying to be clever in one's approach to research it can often overshadow the point that is trying to be made through the text (Foley 1990). I feel it is important that readers, whether they are fellow academics, students, athletes or activists, have a sense of where I am coming from while reading this account, and this is the primary aim of the first chapter.

I was born in a small urban centre in Southern Ontario during the mid-1960s to parents who were employed as teachers at the local high school. There was nothing particularly unusual about my very early childhood until my parents began to worry that I was unable to walk, when many of their friends who had children of the same age had already mastered the skill. My lack of ability in mastering the art of walking led to an appointment at Toronto's sick kids' hospital, where I was diagnosed as having mild cerebral palsy.[3] I was provided with a small brace that had a boot with an iron rod attached to the ankle at either side, which fit into a padded support that fastened around my calf. This little white brace facilitated enough support to enable me, shortly after, to begin walking and running. I wore this brace for a year before I outgrew it and it was replaced by a larger one of a similar style (this time made of brown leather). Much to my delight, by the time I went to kindergarten my right leg was strong enough to support me without the use of the brace, though I wore it to bed for the next year or so.

Some readers might be asking, what do these early memories have to do with an ethnography on the Paralympic Movement? To my mind, the brace is symbolic of difference. I was the only child I knew who wore one. From time to time it marked me out as a figure of ridicule, yet I know other children were teased for all sorts of reasons (and still are, I imagine). However, it was my brace that set me apart. While growing up in elementary and high school I felt that when I was socially shunned it was a result of my impairment, the cerebral palsy rather than any of the other numerous flaws of which I am now only too vividly aware.

From a very early age I have always been fascinated by the act of running, both as an observer who can appreciate the speed at which others run and as a participant. I love to run. The thrill of wind blowing through my hair and the feeling of exhaustion if I push myself too hard. The tingling in my arms as fatigue pulsed through my body. The aching of my lungs as they heave almost uncontrollable in an effort to get more oxygen. These moments, whether in artificial landscapes such as city streets or athletic stadia, or in a more 'natural' environment such as woodlands and other rural settings, were when I really knew I was alive. In the 1970s, however, the act of running was at one and the same time both more and less constrained than it is today. There certainly was a freedom from covert consumerism, in the sense that there were limited products designed specifically for running. Yet running was more physically constraining than it is today. Modern technologies such as Lycra and breathable yet waterproof fabrics had yet to be invented. Running, even as a child and then into my teenage years, was a cumbersome activity during the Southern Ontario winter. Heavy cotton tracksuits often worn under a shell suit that made the wearer feel like a 'boil in the bag' dinner were seldom comfortable. The running 'boom' that resulted from, amongst other things, American Frank Shorter winning the 1972 Munich Olympic Marathon ultimately led to the commercialisation and commodification of running that we see in the first decade of the twenty-first century. In spite of the lack of comfort in running attire during the late 1970s and early 1980s, stories of triumph of great runners from around the world kept the flame of success burning in my mind on many a cold winter's evening. The act of running, despite the odd environmental hardship, captivates my imagination to this day.

These early recollections are in no way unique. Roger Bannister (1955) expressed similar sentiments regarding youthful running in his reflection of his athletic achievement aptly entitled *The First Four Minutes*. There is a freedom in the running one does in childhood, as there is in most playful activities. Success on the athletics track takes a lot more than simple playful running, however. Serious athletic training should be enjoyable, but the structure of training can be intense and it can lead to a particular form of habitus (Howe 2006a; Bale 2004). The embodied nature of training was central to my early understanding of who I was. My father had been a successful local track coach, and his enthusiasm for the sport, which bordered on muscular Christianity, was infectious. Running for me became a game of mimicry, where the goal was to pretend I was one of my father's 'track boys'. Looking back now, it seems like a fanciful world. Growing up in a cultural environment where, in sporting terms, (ice) hockey was celebrated above everything else, I was anomalous. My first sporting heroes were Bill Crothers (Olympic silver medallist) and Bruce Kidd (Commonwealth Champion), who, by the time I remember listening to my father's stories of their prowess, had retired from international athletics. Both of these men had performed valiantly for Canada on the international stage, and I was determined to do the same.

Track and field athletics became the first love of my life, and the middle distances were king. Running both the 800 m and the mile at my primary school with little structured training and even less success did nothing to dampen the enthusiasm. By the time I reached high school I was training four to five times a week, under the supervision of my father, and slowly began to have limited success. Physically, I was not like the other boys I competed against. Born with mild cerebral palsy, the right side of my body is congenitally impaired, which in part hindered my progress as a runner. This impairment takes the form of a mild paralysis, which is referred to medically as hemiplegia. It took longer to learn many physical skills, and because of its relative simplicity and my father's love for athletics I was drawn to running. Being born with hemiplegia, to caring parents, meant that my father spent an hour a day manipulating and massaging my right arm and leg in order to stimulate muscle development and function. The exercise regime undertaken by my father was instrumental in allowing me to run as 'normally' as possible. In my mind I was (and often still am) as graceful as Sebastian Coe and as powerful as Steve Ovett, but in reality I have never been an elegant runner. Throwing myself into the sport, from time to time I was ridiculed for my zest and enthusiasm and no doubt for the ungainly manner in which I ran. Both the act of running and my impairment made me liminal to the social world at high school (Turner 1967). In a sense, I was marginalised both by my impairment and by my consuming desire to run fast. My impairment made me stand out in a small town where difference was considered undesirable. As a response to my marginal status, I threw myself further into world of track and field athletics in an attempt to escape. This strategy worked, and the body culture surrounding my high-school track and field team became a social alternative to the mainstream. The habituation that repetitive running caused made track the primary focus in my life. My only concern was to run well for my family and Canada in the Olympics!

Reality has a way of kicking dreams into touch, and by the time I went to university I had realised that my mortal engine (Hoberman 1992) was so 'flawed' that my dreams of becoming an Olympian were unattainable. The stories of Murray Halberg (Gilmour 1963), who became the Olympic Champion over 5000 m in Rome 1960 in spite of having a 'withered' left arm, had led me to dream throughout high school, but my results never justified my dreaming, and as high school ended I realised that the best I could do was be a bit-part player in provincial championships in my senior year in both cross country and indoor track. Disappointment in myself and dissatisfaction with my (im)perfect body was short-lived. I became aware of competitive opportunities for athletes with cerebral palsy through the Cerebral Palsy International Sport and Recreation Association (CP-ISRA), and increased my training to thirteen times a week in the hope of securing selection for the Canadian team.

Impaired body as the key to the field

After representing Canada at a dual meet against the United States during the summer of 1985, the following year I was selected to represent Canada at the CP-ISRA World Championships in Belgium. Having just finished my first year of a BSc degree in anthropology, I was keen to explore some of the principles and concepts of my studies. Primarily, I was interested in determining whether my participation in this sporting event would be applicable for the recording of field notes – the primary source of data that had been traditionally used by social/cultural anthropologists. I was uncertain of this method of collecting data in this cultural context for a number of reasons. First, the examples of research that were highlighted as good ethnography in first-year anthropology were rather more 'exotic' that this. The Dobi Kung of the African desert and the Yanomamo of the Amazonian rainforest were the two prominent examples. Both of these groups had distinctive cosmologies that made them highly appropriate for the development of early understanding of all things anthropological (see Lee 1979; Chagnon 1983). The second important factor was that I had little awareness or understanding of how and what I should be recording in my field notes. In a sense I began my investigation devoid of any methodological training, which was created both by a degree of apprehension as well as by a thirst for the knowledge of how field notes could produce a useful source of data.

This early training in the method of 'in at the deep end' served me well, as I later went on to my Masters and PhD in the same discipline, and the only prescriptive research training I received was a reading course during my Masters where we systematically went through the book *Ethnography: Principles in Practices* (Hammersley and Atkinson 1989). In other words, during the summer of 1986, when I began the task of recording data on my sporting experiences in field notebooks, I had only read a small number of ethnographies and so my sojourn was an adventure both in a sporting sense and as a 'voyage' of anthropological discovery.

I was determined to make the most of my membership of the Canadian track and field athletics team as an opportunity for fieldwork, and as a result I dutifully collected notes as a member of the team from that summer. Returning to the notes years later, the observations recorded are both useful as well as heavily inscribed with naivety. The naivety is perhaps not unexpected. Since this original sojourn I have attempted systematically to take notes whenever in the company of elite athletes with a disability and the administrative entourage that continues to follow in their wake. In essence, then, this is a multi-site ethnographic study. As I developed as a student of anthropology, the ability to interpret the cultural milieu surrounding sport for the disabled expanded. By 1992, when I began my PhD study on the social implications of the professionalisation of sports medicine in the context of Welsh rugby (see Howe 2001, 2004a), I was still an active member of the Canadian Paralympic team and continued to record notes at national training camps and international events.

In 1996, after over a decade competing internationally, it was important to me to give something back to the sport of athletics, and so I stood as athletes' representative to the International Paralympic Committee Athletics Committee (IPCAC). On becoming an athletes' representative, I was empowered (or so I believed at the time) to help move the sport forward, and though at times this involvement was frustrating I gained access to the techno-political decisions that were made on behalf of the athletes in the sport of track and field athletics. Insight into the political working of an International Paralympic Committee (IPC) technical committee reaffirmed to me that, in spite of the political rhetoric that the organisation was 'athlete centred', there had been a marked shift away from the concerns of some of the athletes, and athletes were by and large absent from the decision-making process. In the past two decades the Paralympic Movement has seen its political environment change most dramatically. The cultural politics of the International Organisations of Sport for the Disabled (IOSD), which is a collective of disability-specific federations – namely the Cerebral Palsy International Sport and Recreation Association (CP-ISRA), the International Blind Sport Association (IBSA), the International Sports Federation for Persons with Intellectual Disability (INAS-FID) and the International Wheelchair and Amputee Sport Association (IWAS)[4] – has been a fruitful area for anthropological investigation. Since the inception of the IPC in 1989, this institution has led to a shift from a participatory model of sport for the disabled to one based on high performance that has been further transformed recently by the IPC's desire to sell their Games and Championships as sporting spectacles.

The desire of the IPC to sell its products creates tension between it and the IOSDs, and as an athlete, administrator and journalist I have been uniquely placed to document this ongoing political battle. This monograph is an ethnographic exploration that adopts the concept of body culture (Brownell 1995) as the nexus between the physical embodiment of athletes with a disability and the structures imposed upon them in light of the development of institutions which govern Paralympic sport. It is a traditional ethnographic monograph in the same vein as the work of Armstrong (1998), Brownell (1995), Klein (1993) and Wacquant (2004) – scholars who have used this model within the sub-discipline of the anthropology of sport. As such, my body was physically present at all of the first-hand observations made here. In fact, my body acted as my first 'gatekeeper' into the world of high-performance sport for the disabled. As previously mentioned, I was an athlete involved in Paralympic athletics. In essence, this volume is about the power relations that have developed in the Paralympic Movement over the past two decades. My position in this work is a result of my habituation as an athlete as much as it is about me as an academic, and because of that I can be seen to be literally running through it. Ultimately, this book is about a distinctive culture that has shaped disabled bodily practice at both a structural level as well as the level of individual identity. What follows are extracts from field notes that highlight that Paralympic sport has come of age. The Paralympic Games are a relatively high-profile mediated event which, at least on the surface, is good for the disabled communitas. As such, the notes will set the stage for the remainder of this study.

Sydney, Australia – 22 October 2000
This evening there was a classic confrontation on the track at Stadium Australia. After the media frenzy of the Olympic Games, the Paralympics

are producing their own drama. Unlike twenty years ago, a large collection of the world's press are present and tonight one of the blue ribbon events of the athletics programme, the women's 800 m wheelchair final, was taking place. The 800 m women's wheelchair (and for that matter the men's 1500 m wheelchair) race have a special place in the history and development of high-performance sport for the disabled. Since 1984, these events have held demonstration status at the Olympic Games. By 1993, the International Association of Athletics Federations (IAAF) had included these events as demonstrations in their bi-annual world championships. These two wheelchair races have done a great deal to showcase the ability of Paralympians. Performances produced by the athletes involved are superior in terms of time achieved for the distance in comparison to ambulant Olympians. People who otherwise would know little about the achievements of elite athletes with a disability get to see these races as part of the media bonanza that is the calling card of the Olympic Movement – a slick, awe-inspiring fortnight of high-energy media production that surrounds the world's most influential sporting spectacle.

For the first time, the Olympic and Paralympic Games were marketed to the world as a single entity. The enthusiasm for the Paralympics has been great, with over a million tickets sold across all venues. This evening, the Australian Paralympic team's answer to Cathy Freeman, Louise Sauvage, is racing over 800 m, and, as with Freeman, Australia expects. Sauvage has been so dominant in women's wheelchair racing that since 1993 that she has won every IAAF demonstration event, and the 1996 and 2000 Olympic demonstration as well. The event today was destined to be another reaffirmation of her physical superiority over the other elite women. Having won the Olympic demonstration weeks earlier in Sydney, the Paralympic outing would be a wheel in the park.

The most captivating quality of sport is its ability to surprise. In the 800 m, this evening, eight of the world's most talented women's wheelchair racers compete in a keenly contested final. Powerful torsos were draped in the latest Lycra racing gear in a rainbow of national colours. From the waist up, these athletes are as chiselled as any on the planet. This is definitely not an event for the light-hearted. Rivalry here is a vicious as anywhere in sport. On the first lap there was some jostling, as can be expected in all 800 m races, and this is one of the reasons that the International Paralympic Committee (IPC) stipulates that wheelchair races that are not run in lanes (800 m–marathon) require all athletes to wear a helmet. So the physical nature of this race was not unexpected.

Down the back straight there was an accident that occurred behind the leading athletes, including Sauvage. There was another surprise for the partisan crowd. Canadian Chantel Petitclerc soundly defeated Sauvage. Petitclerc, a vastly experienced athlete, had seldom managed to get the better of Sauvage, and never until this point on the world stage. Sauvage had finished second. The look of despair on her face was evidence of how much the defeat hurt. In contrast, the celebration of Petitclerc conveyed a delight at realising a dream. In tomorrow's paper, Petitclerc will be quoted as saying 'I dream about Louise more than I do my boyfriend',[5] and this gives some idea how much this victory meant to her.

The drama did not stop there. The host nation was not happy. Australia filed a protest to have the race re-run because one of their athletes, Holly Ladmore, had been involved in the crash. Race referees disqualified Ireland's Patrice Dockery for leaving her lane before the break in the back straight, and the race is set to be re-run in a few days time. Outraged Canadian officials appealed the decision to re-run the race, knowing full well that the Australian protested because Sauvage had lost the race. Canada appealed, citing the fact that the crash had occurred behind the chief protagonists. A long and frustrating debate ensued into the small hours of the next morning. Canada's appeal was ultimately upheld, and the result was confirmed as official.

The result of the women's 800 m at the Sydney Paralympic Games can be seen as a watershed for several reasons. Athletic rivalries were centre-stage at the Paralympics, and such rivalries are often seen as a hallmark of professional sport (Whannel 1992; Smart 2005). As a rivalry, Petitclerc and Sauvage fit into the classic mould made famous in middle-distance terms by Sebastian Coe and Steve Ovett, most notably in the lead-up to the 1980 Moscow Olympics: Petitclerc small and graceful, not unlike Coe, and Sauvage a powerhouse with immense physical talent, one of the chief ingredients attributed to the success of Ovett. After the surprise victory by Petitclerc, Sauvage continued to have success on the IAAF stage, winning demonstration events in both 2001 and 2003. Petitclerc proved to herself and her fans at the 2002 Commonwealth Games that her victory over Sauvage in Sydney two years earlier was not a flash in the pan. The Manchester Commonwealth Games marked another crucial development in Paralympic sport. Petitclerc, Sauvage, Grey-Thompson and others in the women's wheelchair 800 m were, for the first time at a mainstream athletics event, competing in an event that had full medal status. After the second victory over Sauvage, Petitclerc was clear that it was the status of the race that was the real achievement. 'It is a very special medal. No matter who might have won this gold medal, it would have been an historic occasion' (Kalbfuss 2002). Without question this victory in Manchester was a personal achievement for Petitclerc, but the historical importance of the recognition of the elite status of wheelchair athletes is perhaps more significant.

Readers are likely to recognise the image of Paralympic sport highlighted above, and many may expect this book to be a celebration of ability rather than a discussion about disability – and in an odd way it is. There is much to celebrate in what the public sees of the Paralympics. Athletes with a disability are performing magnificent feats, with their bodies trained to their peak, and continually searching for more. Multinational sponsors are now commonplace at the Paralympic Games, but, as with all sporting practices, there is another less desirable dimension to this sporting phenomenon that is, I believe, a cultural struggle that is a direct result of commercialisation of the Paralympic sporting practice. The development of a 'thick description' of the cultural environment surrounding the Paralympic Movement requires the anthropologist to articulate his position theoretically. In order that this may be exposed, this monograph adopts a historical materialist account of sport for the disabled and its primary flagship, Paralympic sport. Adoption of this approach, which is philosophically linked to Marxist social theory, highlights explanations that focus upon the economic and social environment that surround sport for the disabled and how these practices do not in many cases match the public perceptions of the Movement. Following Gleeson (1997: 184), it is clear that a materialist analysis of sport for the disabled is paramount:

> The political implications of dematerialising the explanation of disability are clear. The view of disability as an attitudinal structure and/or aesthetic construct avoids the issue of how these ideological realities are formed. Idealist prescriptions are consequently reduced either to the ineffectual realm of 'attitude changing' policies or the oppressive suggestion that disabled people should conform to aesthetic and behavioural 'norms' in order to qualify for social approbation.

In essence, Paralympic sport is no different from Olympic or other forms of what Bale (2004) has called achievement sport. As such, Paralympic sport has its positive as well as its negative attributes. All too often sport for the disabled is portrayed as innocent and pure – perhaps this is because the mainstream believes that a disability makes someone virtuous or rather that, because sport for the disabled is something 'given' to the disabled communitas, it must be a good thing. Whatever the reason, I am hopeful that this monograph will allow readers the opportunity to critically evaluate the Paralympic sporting practice in the manner they would any other cultural environment under investigation.

The structure of the book

This monograph is divided into two major parts. The first of these, entitled 'Sport and disability', focuses upon the structural nature of the Paralympic Movement. This section opens in Chapter 2 with a brief social history of sport for the disabled. Included are developments through Stoke Mandeville Hospital and the desire in the post-war West to use sport as a vehicle for rehabilitation toward normality. Different sporting organisations for the disabled will be explored, while emphasis is placed on how their development has 'served' these distinctive populations. A discussion of how and why the International Paralympic Committee (IPC) was established will draw this chapter to a close. Effectively, the social historical account will end when I enter the field in the mid-1980s, since this monograph has a strong diachronic element. Chapter 3 provides what I have called a 'lived history', a distillation of field notes from the mid-1980s until the present, which will allow the reader to establish and understand the progress or otherwise of the cultural politics of the Paralympic Movement as directly experienced by the author.

Chapter 4 starts by exploring the politics of disability. This is followed by a discussion of the Foucauldian concept of governmentality that is a way into the political world of classification within sport for the disabled. A struggle over the classification process highlights the power imbalance between the IOSDs and the IPC. This imbalance has led to the transformation of elite sporting provision for the disabled. Important in this discussion will be an exploration of both the medical and the social models of disability, and how the debates surrounding these models within disability studies can be used to facilitate an understanding of the social firmament that surrounds the classification systems used within sport for the disabled. The tools that the IPC employs to control the federations will be examined, illuminating the desire of the IPC to mirror the developments in the IOC. Currently the IPC is considered to be a part of the Olympic 'family', but whether this association has a positive impact on the disabled sporting communitas will be determined in this chapter.

Chapter 5 examines the impact of the media spotlight on the development of the Paralympic Games as a sporting spectacle. Attention will be paid to the positive impact of media coverage upon society in terms of education of the public with regard to difference. Media focus can have a negative impact, as the media does not always accurately represent the Paralympic subculture. The resulting coverage can play a role in further segregating Paralympians from the mainstream high-performance sporting communitas.

The second part of the monograph is entitled 'Impairment, sport and performance', which will be distinguished using the body and the concept of embodiment as the site of the cultural investigation into sport for the disabled. Chapter 6 opens this section by highlighting scholarship that illuminates the importance of exploring bodily culture. Drawing on structural issues highlighted in Part 1, this chapter will explore how issues related to classification (on one level a structural issue), which makes sport for the disabled so distinctive, create a paradox between the necessity for sport to be about enhanced human performance on one hand and the use of imperfect vessels (the body) to portray this on the other. Following on from this, Chapter 7 discusses the technological improvements in wheelchairs and prosthetic limbs. This will be used to shed light on how this technology is being used to improve performances of elite disabled athletes, but at the same time is a vehicle for the increased marginalisation of the impaired bodies these technologies are designed to 'assist'. Finally, whether the advances in technology are actually of benefit to the cause of empowering disabled athletes, and the disabled communitas at large, will be considered.

Chapter 8 explores how the practice of sport with ever increasing 'opportunities' for the impaired has resulted in certain types of bodies being eliminated from the media spotlight and, to some degree, removed from internationally viable sporting programmes. While these individuals still have a competitive sporting outlet within their impairment-specific federations, the fear is that the definition of an athlete with a disability is getting more visibly 'normal'. How the Paralympic Movement can reverse this trend and what steps can be taken in the future in order to guarantee equity of opportunity for all disabled athletes are important questions that will be addressed using the case study of the integration of the Paralympic Programme into Athletics Canada.

The book concludes with an exploration of the use of ethnographic methods in an appendix entitled *Through an Anthropological Lens*.

Part 1
Sport and disability

2   A social history of sport for the disabled

A comprehensive history of sport for the disabled has yet to be written, and, as an anthropologist, it would be remiss to suggest that a single chapter in a monograph might achieve this aim. No doubt such a project requires a volume of its own. It is important, however, for this monograph to highlight significant trends and 'moments' in the history of the Paralympic Movement as well as more broadly within sport for the disabled. There can, of course, be difficulties with writing a 'potted' history. Importantly, this chapter must be seen as an ethnocentric account of the history of sport for the disabled since the story that unfolds within it is laden with a heavy Western bias. Records appear to show that organised sport for the disabled communitas was a Western advent (as in fact were many of the sporting practices that are commonplace today), but that does not mean that elsewhere in the world sport as we understand it was not being practised. Documentation surrounding the early development of sport for the disabled appears to point to a Western development (DePauw and Gavron 1995 [2005]) and, more specifically, a beginning in the United Kingdom during the final stages of the Second World War (Goodman 1986; Scruton 1998).

On a very basic level there appear to have been three stages in the development of sporting provision for the disabled. In the first instance, provision was designed to aid in the *rehabilitation* of individuals who were seriously injured during the Second World War. This research, however, was not simply interested in the act of rehabilitation. Following Seymour (1998: xiv–xv),

> the word 'rehabilitation' has been appropriated by medicine and the rehabilitation industry, the concept of rehabilitation employed in this study relates to broader issues of embodiment which may take place in contexts far removed from the agencies and auspices of conventional rehabilitation.

The use of physical activity and, more explicitly, sport in the act of rehabilitation was a novel concept in the 1940s (Guttmann 1976). It was felt that sport, along with arts and crafts, was an important vehicle into a productive life (Scruton 1998; Anderson 2003). Second, sport for the disabled was about *participation*, and as a result a number of International Organisations of Sport for the Disabled (IOSD) were formed to enable athletes from around the world to compete in sport alongside their physical equals. These organisations were structured around particular impairment groups (spinal cord injuries, where individuals were often confined[1] to a wheelchair; visually impaired; hearing impaired;[2] cerebral palsy; and amputees). The IOSDs introduced systems that were designed to create a level playing field by establishing distinctive classification systems for each impairment group. Third, in light of these developments a focus upon *high performance* ultimately led to the establishment of the International Paralympic Committee (IPC) in Düsseldorf on 21 September 1989, and officially began what is commonly referred to as the Paralympic Movement.

An exploration of significant historical milestones in the development of sport for the disabled is undertaken in this chapter, including developments through Stoke Mandeville Hospital and the desire in the post-war West to use sport as a vehicle for rehabilitation toward normality. This is followed by a brief chronology of events that led to the development of the different sporting organisations for the disabled. Of importance is the emphasis placed on how development of the IOSDs has 'served' distinctive populations.

Very brief histories of the Paralympic Movement highlight a common development as follows.

In 1944, Sir Ludwig Guttmann established a spinal cord injury unit at Stoke Mandeville Hospital in Aylesbury, England. To coincide with the Olympics in London during 1948, he launched the first Stoke Mandeville Games that same year. It has been suggested that it was Guttmann's vision to stage a Games festival every four years in the same city as the Olympics. During 1952 the Games were held at Stoke Mandeville again (rather than Helsinki host city of the Olympics), and in part because of this those in attendance established the International Stoke Mandeville Games Federation (ISMGF) to coordinate the staging of future events. It was not until 1960 that the Games were held outside England, and it was this event in Rome that is generally seen as the first Paralympic Games.

The prefix 'para' within the term 'Paralympic Movement' means 'alongside'. Rome 1960 is considered to have been the first Paralympics because it was the first full-scale event to run in the same country at the same time as the Olympics. The term 'Paralympic', however, was not used until 1964 in Tokyo.

As the IPC website states,

The word 'Paralympic' derives from the Greek preposition 'para' ('beside' or 'alongside') and the word 'Olympics', the Paralympics being the parallel Games to the Olympics. The word 'Paralympic' was originally a pun combining 'paraplegic' and 'Olympic', however with the inclusion of other disability groups and close associations with the Olympic Movement, it now represents 'parallel' and 'Olympic' to illustrate how the two movements exist side by side.[3]

However, such histories fail to give much insight into how sport became important within the disabled communitas. It is the social significance of sport in the rehabilitation of the disabled to which we shall now turn our attention.

Sport as a means to an end

Much has been written about the way the disabled communitas has been oppressed by the institution of medicine (see Chapter 4). Social theorists of disability, following the lead of Oliver (1990) have discussed how the disabled communitas has been marginalised because such impairments are seen as medical rather than social problems. The link between medicine and disability can be seen to be extremely robust with regard to the early development of sporting provision for the disabled, in part because of the desire to improve physical performance.

Stoke Mandeville Hospital was built as an EMS (Emergency Medical Services) Hospital in 1940, and it was here that Dr Ludwig Guttmann, a neurosurgeon, arrived in 1944 and was asked to help rehabilitate spinal cord injured ex-servicemen. These men were kept in separate wards, as they were seen as a different type of medical patients:

> [I]n the early stages of World War II spinal cord casualties were segregated in special units – the view being that there would be better chances there for adequate treatment than could be given in general medical, surgical, orthopaedic, or neurosurgical wards.
>
> (Scruton 1998: 11)

Segregated and with time on their hands, these men were forced to entertain themselves. Doing his rounds, Guttmann saw a group of patients frantically moving in their wheelchairs outside the dormitory blocks using a puck and an upside-down walking stick. These simple actions led to the development of what was referred to as 'wheelchair polo' (Goodman 1986). This game was a big draw for the patients, but polo was replaced first by netball and then by basketball (Scruton 1998: 27–28) because the use of the 'stick' at the same time as propelling the wheelchair was an overtly dangerous activity.

Exercise in the form of sport became a staple in the rehabilitation program of all the patients. As Scruton (1998: 14) suggested:

> Before a patient in the National Spinal Injuries Centre graduates from the Physiotherapy Department, he is now expected to dress himself in a few minutes, to maintain an upright position without artificial support of any kind, to get himself in and out of bed unaided, to walk on crutches, know how to swim and to have developed into an all round paraplegic sportsman.

The aim of the rehabilitation was not the pursuit of physical excellence that is the hallmark of the Paralympic Games today, but rather a desire to get these men back into work and paying taxes: 'It was not the physical prowess of the disabled ex-servicemen and women that mattered, but whether or not their stay at the Unit culminated in "useful" employment' (Anderson 2003: 462).

The embodiment of the employment-driven ethos of Stoke Mandeville Hospital can be seen in Guttmann's initiation and continual publishing of *The Cord* from 1947. *The Cord* was basically a lifestyle magazine that Guttmann established, to be written and edited by paraplegics, although he himself became the most active contributor and essentially it became a vehicle for his gospel (Goodman 1986: 129). It was in this publication that ex-servicemen and women could learn about how others who had suffered a spinal cord injury were able to deal with daily activities as well as psychologically adjusting to their change in physical circumstances.

Guttmann wrote an article for *The Cord* in 1948 entitled 'Readjustment to a New Psychological Aspects':

> When the body is shattered and thrown out of gear by a disaster of such magnitude as a spinal cord injury, it is inevitable that the mind, too, falls into chaos. The will to live, despite great physical handicap, has to be restored, and the patient's full co-operation has to be gained in order to win his mind and heart back to activity and useful work. The ultimate aim is to make him as independent as possible and to restore him to his rightful place in social life.
>
> (quoted in Scruton 1998: 16)

It was the imperative of returning ex-servicemen to a 'normal' social life, particularly as taxpayers, that made sport such an appropriate tool in helping with rehabilitation.

Emphasis on the treatment of individuals injured in the line of national duty no doubt did little to help with the treatment (both physically and emotionally) of those who were congenitally impaired. The Tomlinson Report related to the Disabled Persons (Employment) Act was passed by the British Government in 1944. As a result of the ongoing war with Germany, MPs who were war veterans 'insisted that the act give preference to those injured as a result of war service' (Anderson 2003: 469). In light of this, it is not surprising that development of sporting provision for the disabled focused upon athletes with a spinal cord injury who were based in units reserved, at least in post-war Britain, for ex-service men. It was still a return to work that was the ultimate aim of those working at Stoke Mandeville Hospital. Guttmann stressed the importance of work in *The Cord* in 1948

> If there is any delay in providing the man with a job, or at least in giving him facilities for further vocational training, he may well soon not want to bother about work, will become inactive, and eventually deteriorate into a professional charity case.
>
> (Guttmann 1948: 7, quoted in Anderson 2003: 469)

Rehabilitative sport as a vehicle for getting injured military personnel back to work was the first stage in the development of sport for the disabled. Guttmann's lasting legacy is the fact that physical activity and sport are widely acknowledged to be central to contemporary rehabilitation for traumatic and congenital impairments. The establishment of the Stoke Mandeville Games is another related significant contribution Guttmann made to the practice of sport for the disabled. This development began the sports-participation phase of the Movement.

The rise of the Stoke Mandeville Games

Dr Guttmann was quick to realise that sport for the war wounded was a way of getting the public's attention, stating,

> at the prize-giving ceremony in 1949, I was somewhat carried away by the success of the Games that year and I dared to express the hope that the time might come when the event would be truly international and the Stoke Mandeville Games would achieve world fame as the disabled man and women's equivalent of the Olympic Games.
>
> (quoted in Goodman 1986: 150)

It was only a year prior to that, on 28 July 1948, the day of the London Olympics opening ceremony, that the first Stoke Mandeville Games took place. This shows a clear vision of the future and the value that sport could play in the lives of the disabled. Writing in his *Textbook of Sport for the Disabled* (1976), Guttmann highlights the importance of the rehabilitative qualities of sport

> The immense value of sport in the physical, psychological and social rehabilitation of these most severely physically handicapped patients was recognised and became the incentive to many of them to carry on with their sporting activities after discharge from hospital and to become true sportsmen and sportswomen in their own right. Clinical sport is now widely used and has gained its secure place in the field of sport.
>
> (Guttmann 1976: 3)

In spite of the rather dated terminology (e.g. the use of the word 'handicap'), this is a relatively functionalist account of the role that sport can play in the life of the disabled population. Guttmann believed the ethos of sport could also be good for the improvement of the individual:

> In training, one is engaged in the first place in self-struggle, with a desire to promote the best abilities and talents one is able to develop in oneself. In this struggle, by obeying the rules of sport, moral qualities, such as self-confidence, initiative, courage and endurance, self-discipline and fairness as well as team spirit, comradeship and friendship, are developed. These are

the virtues which distinguish the real sportsman from a man whose motivation is simply to practise physical exercises for health reasons.

(Guttmann 1976: 10)

These moral qualities would not seem out of place in the rhetoric that surrounds the ethical studies of sporting practice today (Simon 1991; Loland 2002), though their literal existence may be continually questioned by those interested in the social importance of sporting practice and that are not aligned with the functionalist school. As if to highlight this fact, Guttmann suggests that 'any exaggerated nationalism, commercialism, or political, racial and religious discrimination is quite inconsistent with the ideals of the Games and would be abhorrent' (Guttmann 1976: 33).

By the 1956 Olympic Games the ISMGF had received the Fearnley Cup for 'outstanding achievement in the service of the Olympic ideals' (Guttmann 1976: 32). It may have been the developments within ISMGF that led to this recognition and enabled the Games to take place in Rome – the same city as the Olympics – in 1960. At this point the ideals of the International Stoke Mandeville Games Federation (ISMGF) were said to have been embodied in the symbol of three entwining wheels that represented friendship, unity and sportsmanship (Guttmann 1976). It is with these ideals in mind that this chapter turns to historical snapshots of the Paralympic Games over a forty-year period that highlight key changes in the Movement.

Historical snapshots – the Paralympic Games (1960–2000)

Rome 1960

The Games held in Rome in 1960 have gone down in history as the first Paralympic Games, though the term 'Paralympic' was not officially recognised by the IOC until it was used to describe the 1988 Games in Seoul (Doll-Tepper 1999). Rome hosted the Olympic Games in 1960, and Sir Ludwig Guttmann was influential in paving the way for the Paralympics to follow directly on from the Olympics. Guttmann had become acquainted with an Italian Professor, Antonia Maglio, through his long-term research into spinal cord injuries. Maglio had, like Guttmann, run a research centre focusing on impairment. Guttmann and Maglio decided it would increase the profile of the International Stoke Mandeville Games if they were held in Rome shortly after the Olympics. These Games were held without modern consideration for accessibility, and athletes who attended confirm that the military were quite useful in carrying them up and down flights of stairs. Since all previous Games had been held at Stoke Mandeville, issues of accessibility had been less acute – at least on first sight.

In Rome, many events were held within the confines of the village; however, two sports that later became flagship events at the Paralympic Games, basketball and athletics, needed additional facilities. This required the development of an accessible transportation system. The Games were held on 19–24 September in association with the Italian Olympic Committee just a week after the conclusion of the XVII Olympic Summer Games. Involvement of the Italian Olympic Committee was indeed progress, since it highlighted the acceptance, at least in Italy, of the fledgling Paralympic Movement. It would be another four decades before such an association became formalised during the Sydney Games of 2000. Over 300 athletes from twenty-three countries took part in this event, which drew some 5000 spectators to the opening ceremony. Still today, the best attended events during the Paralympic Games are the opening and closing ceremonies.

Events, that were not necessarily deemed to have a therapeutic value, included an adapted version of the modern pentathlon (archery, swimming, javelin, shot put and club throw), as well as archery as a single event and table tennis (both single and doubles). While these Games were just for wheelchair athletes, two things were established: first, a desire for an international sporting festival for the disabled to follow on from the Olympic Games; and second, a realisation that in order to successfully achieve this aim the physical environment must be accessible to the disabled population. At the closing ceremony, Guttmann was described by Pope John XXIII as the 'de Coubertin of the Paralyzed' (Scruton 1998: xiii). More importantly, Guttmann stated at the time:

> It can now be concluded that the first experiment to hold the Stoke Mandeville Games as an entity in another country, as an international sports festival comparable with the Olympic Games and other international sporting events for the abled-bodied has been highly successful.
>
> (Scruton 1998: 310)

Tokyo 1964

The success of the Games in Rome was enough to get the Paralympic Movement rolling. Guttmann felt that, to increase the profile of the International Stoke Mandeville Games, they must follow the Olympics to the Japanese capital of Tokyo. Japanese observers at the Rome Games spoke admiringly about events in Italy, and this enabled Guttmann and the International Stoke Mandeville Games Committee (which he led) to establish a working relationship with counterparts in Japan. A Japanese medical researcher, Dr Nakamura, visited Guttmann at the hospital at Stoke Mandeville and at the Wheelchair Games at the same venue in 1962, to which the Japanese sent two athletes. The following year Dr Nakamura brought along a team of specialists in spinal cord injuries. Travelling with this group was Mr Kasai, who was the Chair of the recently developed Japanese Sports Association for the Disabled (JSAD), which had close ties with the Japanese Government. Because of his influence within broader Japanese society, Mr Kasai was an ideal figure to chair the organisation of the 1964 Paralympic Games. Through the influence of Kasai, funding of the Games came, for the first time, from a mix of public and private sector sources.

The opening and closing ceremonies once again drew the biggest crowds (approximately 5000 spectators each), and were held in the presence of Japanese Royalty in the form of His Imperial Highness Prince Akahito and Princess Michiko. This helped to lift the profile of the event, with a degree of national media interest. The Games themselves were also larger, with a total of 375 athletes (307 men) from twenty-one countries. For the first time athletes at these Games competed in track races (over 60 m), and so this was the beginning of what was to become the most colourful sport in the Paralympic programme. This event and the development of racing wheelchair technology (see Chapter 7) helped to increase the profile of athletes who used wheelchairs, though at this juncture it was only paraplegic athletes who were eligible to compete. At the end of the Games a meeting was held, and the International Sport Organisation for the Disabled (ISOD) was formed to administer events for athletes with physical and sensory impairments. In other words, this group was designed to service other disability groups that were outside the remit of the ISMGF. It was at these Games that the term 'Paralympics' was first used (DePauw and Gavron 1995), though there is some confusion in the historical record as to whether the term initially meant 'paraplegic' or 'parallel' Olympics (Mason 2002: 118).

Tel Aviv 1968

In an ideal world, the next Games would have been held in Mexico City. In spite of the enthusiasm of Mexican officials present during the Games in Tokyo with a view to hosting the event immediately after the Olympics, the Mexican Government announced in 1966 that it would not be hosting the Paralympics, citing technical difficulties within the organisational process. This 'rejection' of the Olympic host was certainly a blow to the agenda of Guttmann and those involved in promoting sport for the disabled on the international stage. The Israeli Government, lobbied by the ILAN Society (a group of disability activists), offered to host the International Stoke Mandeville Games in 1968 just outside Tel Aviv. The opening ceremony held on 4 November at Jerusalem's Hebrew University was attended by 10 000 people, and events got underway in the presence of the Deputy Prime Minister, Mr Yigal Allon.

Once again the Games expanded, with 750 athletes from twenty-nine countries taking part. Compared with 1964, the sporting programme had also become more comprehensive: lawn bowls, basketball for women, weightlifting and a 100m wheelchair sprint were added. In spite of being pushed to one side by the organising nation of the Olympic Games, there was enough interest from around the world for another nation to be eager to host the Games in four years' time.

The year 1968 saw the dawn of the International Special Olympics, which is only worth mentioning because athletes who have been involved in the Paralympics are often misrepresented as 'Special Olympians'. Athletes involved in the International Special Olympics are not involved in high-performance sport (much like many of those involved with the ISOD or the ISMGF prior to 1988). However, the Special Olympics is a universal movement that helps those with intellectual disabilities to stay physically active (Mosher 1991). Today Paralympians have a distinctive attitude to training and preparation that aligns them with their able-bodied counterparts, except perhaps for the quantifiable quality of their performances. This year also saw the formation of the International Cerebral Palsy Society, which in 1978 established the Cerebral Palsy International Sport and Recreation Association (CP-ISRA). The CP-ISRA was established to provide an outlet for the participation of people with cerebral palsy in international sporting events. It was not until 1980, however, that athletes with cerebral palsy were part of the Paralympic Games.

Heidelberg 1972

While the III Paralympic Games were not held in the same city as the summer Olympics, they were held in the same nation. With the help of the German Disabled Sports Association (DVS), the International Stoke Mandeville Games Organising Committee had agreed to hold the Games in Munich after the Olympics had left the city; however, the organisers of the Munich Olympics, in an attempt to offset the cost of hosting the Games, had decided to sell off the athletes' village as flats at the conclusion of the Games. The DVS tried in vain to locate alternative accommodation, but such was the success of the developing movement there was nowhere in the city appropriate to house 1000 competitors.

Fortunately the city of Heidelberg suggested that the Games use the city's university, and in particular the Institute of Physical Training. With generous support from the Federal Government as well as the regional authorities (Baden-Württemberg) and the National Olympic Committee, the DVS was able to run a highly successful Games. The President of the Federal Republic of Germany, Dr Gustav Heineman, opened the Games on 2 August, and just over 1000 athletes representing forty-one countries were present. As well as the largest number of athletes so far, the German Games were a watershed for another important reason, as athletes with visual impairments were included for the first time.

The inclusion of visually-impaired athletes in the programme, even in a demonstration capacity, sparked a re-think in the organisation of sport for the disabled. In particular, after the Games the coaches and officials suggested that rules for each sport should be officially codified, and committees were established to remove the burden of responsibility from the Games technical committee. Codification of the rules and regulations of Paralympic sport may be seen as the first of many steps from the participation model to the high-performance model of sport for the disabled. It has been argued that the creation of these committees 'led to more self-determination in the Movement, especially in the development of wheelchair sports'.[4] Of course this 'self-determination' was led by the organisers and not by the athletes, which means that while the Games may have had self-determination, it was not the athletes that had responsibility for this (Howe and Jones 2006). Also of note is how participation-driven the Games were at this time. The IPC website suggests it was these Games in Germany that supplied the first beer tent, which then became a staple of the entertainment in the village up to and including the 1992 Games. A beer tent within the Games village does not sit easily with the ethos of a high-performance sports event.

Toronto 1976

Toronto played host to the Games in 1976, with forty-two countries and over 1600 athletes in attendance. This event was known either as the *Olympiad for the Physically Disabled* or as the *Torontolympiad* (Legg et al. 2004) in an attempt to make explicit the link with the Olympic Games held in Montreal that year. There were due to be forty-six countries in attendance, but several withdrew from the Games in protest at the involvement of apartheid South Africa. This was the first Games that recognised with full medal status the events for the amputee and visually-impaired athletes. At the Games there were 261 amputee athletes and 187 with visual impairments. Inclusion of two new impairment groups, with their own distinctive classification systems, meant that the logistical issues of organising the Paralympic Games became more complex. From the perspective of organising the competitive schedule, these issues become clear. Not only were there multiple classifications within each disability group, but also, in light of the ethos of participation, many athletes competed in more than one sport. It had not been uncommon, since the first Games staged at Stoke Mandeville in Aylesbury, England, for athletes to compete in more than one sport – for example, athletes would swim, do athletics and play basketball at the same Games. By 1976, with the addition of the visually impaired and amputee athletes who also embodied the 'have a go' sporting ethos, the organisation of the competitive schedule had become a mammoth task.

Canadian society was at the time, not unlike all Western nations, not easily accessible for athletes with a disability. Accommodation of competitors with varied disabilities could not or would not be arranged, so all athletes stayed together. The Games were held in the suburb of Etobicoke, and thus the wheelchair athletes stayed at York University, which was relatively close at hand. Competitors from the other disability groups were housed at the University of Toronto or the Ontario Institute for the Blind, both located in the centre of the city at some distance from the competitive venues. The increased complexity of organising a multidisability Paralympic Games facilitated the development of an organisational structure that would allow relatively open communication between the event organisers and the fledging IOSDs. The Canadian organisers managed to drum up media interest in the Games, showing highlights on the publicly-funded TV Ontario, and the opening ceremony again was a major draw, with a reported 24000 spectators attending.

The programme of athletics for athletes in wheelchairs had been expanded to include 200 m, 400 m, 800 m and 1500 m races. For the first time, therefore, the middle distances were included – events that have done so much to highlight the ability of wheelchair racers. These events have since been included as demonstrations on the programme of every Olympic Games since 1984. For the first time, a new sport specially adapted to the athletes with visual impairment was given full medal status. Goalball, as it is known, had been played as a demonstration event in Germany four years earlier. The game is played in a gymnasium using a standard volleyball court, and each team is made up of three players who must wear eye shades so that all are completely blind. Markings on the court are laid out with two layers of duct tape so that the court is tactile to allow the players to get their bearings on court. The idea is to bowl (as in lawn bowls, not 'cricket' style) the ball, which has a bell in it in order to attract the attention of the players. A goal is scored when the ball crosses the line one team is defending.

Including an impairment-specific created game as part of the official Paralympic programme marks a significant point in the development of the Movement. Until now the sporting programme at the Paralympic Games had consisted of events that had been adapted from the mainstream sporting provision. The inclusion of goalball in the Paralympics meant that the Movement was not simply trying to mirror the Olympics but was also attempting to establish distinctive competitive opportunities for its athletes. This year 1976 also marked the beginning of the Winter Paralympic Games, the first being held in Örnsköldsvik, Sweden. While developments within the winter Games are interesting and distinct from the summer variety, a comprehensive understanding of all social/cultural political issues surrounding their development requires separate treatment although many of the central trends are not dissimilar.

Arnhem 1980

The fledgling Movement had been working tirelessly to achieve recognition from the IOC for over twenty years. It was therefore expected that the 1980 Paralympic Games would be held in the same city as the Olympic Games. The ISMGF had attempted to contact the Soviet Government in 1976 in the hope of working alongside them. It has been suggested that Soviet officials 'claimed to not have citizens with disabilities' (Legg et al. 2004: 34), such was the stigma associated with impairments in the eyes of the authorities. This meant that ISMGF had to plan to stage the Games themselves, which arguably was a retrograde step. On the positive side, three nations were eager to play host to the Games. South Africa, which because of its policy of apartheid had caused the withdrawal of several nations from the event in Toronto, was not considered a serious contender. Denmark also expressed interest, but the successful bid went to the Netherlands which, through the Dutch Sports Association for the Disabled, had put together an impressive package. In order to increase awareness and sports for the Games at home, in early 1977 the Dutch established the Foundation of the Olympic Games for the Disabled. Not only was South Africa not awarded the Games; its participation also threatened to derail the whole event, and it were asked not to attend.

Funded by a television bingo programme that was launched on public television in 1976, the Games were held at the National Sports Center in Arnhem, and patronage of the Dutch royal family guaranteed public support. Further support was offered by the military, which provided army facilities to house the athletes and an increasing number of officials. Once again forty-two countries took part, and there were almost 2000 competitors. For the first time, athletes with cerebral palsy took apart. With a fourth disability group, the logistics of running the Games became ever more complex. More than 1000 gold medals were awarded, meaning that on average there was one gold medal for every two competitors. The is a clear indication that these Games were not as competitive as the ones that followed. It is the image created by Games like these and those in 1984 that have had a detrimental impact on the Paralympic Movement today.

Sitting volleyball for amputee athletes made its debut at these Games, and goalball had become so popular there were twelve nations taking part in the Paralympic tournament. Following the success of the visually impaired events at the Games, the IBSA was established in 1981. As a result of the success of the Arnhem Games, and the increased number of groups with a vested interest in the Games, it was clear that the four disability groups needed to work together. The complex nature of the organisation led to the establishment of the International Co-ordinating Committee (ICC) in 1982, a group that had equal representation from each federation (DePauw and Gavron 2005). The four disability-specific federations, namely the Cerebral Palsy International Sports and Recreation Association (CP-ISRA), the International Blind Sports Association (IBSA), the International Sport Organisation for the Disabled (ISOD) and the International Stoke Mandeville Games Federation (ISMGF), came together to form the ICC with the explicit aim of organising the Paralympic Games from 1988 onward. This organisation was by no means democratic. Steadward suggests:

> The ICC was not a democratic organization, did not report to national members, had no constitution and was in fact only an agreement between the four federations. The presidency (pro tem) changed every 6 months or every executive meeting, and decisions had to be taken unanimously.
>
> (1996: 31)

It was this organisation that was to form the template for the International Paralympic Committee (IPC) to be formed at the end of the decade.

Stoke Mandeville, UK and New York, USA 1984

There was a move as early as 1977 to secure the same host city as the Olympics in 1984. With the financial disaster of the 1976 Olympics in Montreal, the IOC was keen to give host nations as big a lead-up to the Games as possible so that they could secure the Olympic Movement's financial future. In hindsight, if the ICC had been more established at that time of the 1984 Paralympics it is likely the Games would have been held in Los Angeles. The independent IOSDs, most of whom were in their infancy, lacked the political understanding and collective voice to impress upon the Los Angeles Olympic Organising Committee (LAOOC) the value of having the Paralympics use the Olympic venues after the Games had closed. Instead the Games were held on two continents, with three disability groups (amputee and les autres,[5] cerebral palsy, and visually impaired) holding their Games in Long Island, New York, and athletes in wheelchairs returning to their spiritual home of Stoke Mandeville.

In spite of a split venue, there were nearly 1800 athletes from forty-five countries competing in New York for competitions from 16 to 30 June, with 900 medals won. These Games were funded through public and private sources, and the media coverage of the Games was the most comprehensive to date – though, it must be said, still a shadow of that achieved by the Olympics in Los Angeles. The major US television networks and newspapers were present, as well as BBC TV, Dutch TV, West German TV and Swedish radio and TV. The US President at the time, Ronald Reagan, officially opened the Games, and throughout the Games more than 80 000 spectators supported the athletes across a total of thirteen events.

Athletes with amputations were able to compete from either a seated position in a wheelchair or a standing position, and as a result the ISOD established a system with nine different classes. Individuals who were managed by the CP-ISRA were organised into eight classes that distinguished athletes by the amount of spasticity they had and in what particular part of the body it was present. The IBSA had decided to class its athletes by the degree of usable vision into three categories, the first having no usable vision and the third having 10 per cent usable vision.

On the other side of the Atlantic, and almost a month later, the British Paraplegic Sports Society (BPSS) organised the Games at the Stoke Mandeville stadium from 22 July until 1 August. Competing there were more than 1100 athletes, who represented forty-one nations over fourteen events. HRH The Prince of Wales opened Games, and for the first time a marathon event was held. The success of these multisite Games was evident in the number of athletes and countries that were able to attend events on both sides of the Atlantic. Overall, some 2900 athletes were involved. Those in charge of organising both events did realise that in future it might be prudent, in part due to economies of scale, that the Games be a coordinated effort. This would help nations to fund teams to attend the Games, rather than having to split their resources by sending smaller outfits to various locations. It would also enable the ICC to establish a single message to possible host cities with regard to the nature of the ability of (dis)abled athletes. By 1986 a fifth group would also be involved in deliberation; the International Sports Federation for Persons with Mental Handicap (INAS-FMH). This would later become part of the

Paralympic family, when its athletes attended the Games in Atlanta in 1996. The INAS-FMH[6] was established as an organisation to facilitate high-performance sport opportunities for athletes with intellectual disabilities, thus making it distinct from the Special Olympics.

The biggest positive step that arose out of the attempts to have the Paralympics in Los Angeles following the Olympic Games was that two wheelchair races were given demonstration status within the Olympics athletics programme. The 800 m open wheelchair race for women and 1500 m open wheelchair race for men have been demonstration events during every Olympiad since Los Angeles, and have arguably done more to raise awareness of the ability of (dis)abled athletes than any other in the history of sport for the disabled. At this time there was a push to have athletes with a disability included in the Olympic Games of the future. The establishment of the Commission for the Inclusion of Athletes with a Disability (CIAD) was formed to place pressure on the IOC to include more Paralympic events in future programmes. Steadward (1996: 36–37), then the first president of the IPC stated,

> There is certainly no doubt that the [wheelchair men's 1500 m and women's 800 m] demonstration events included in the past Olympic Games have stimulated both public and athlete interest but the ultimate experience in competitive sport is still the quest for the Olympic gold medal. It is the quest for full medal status that CIAD now pursues.

The push for further inclusion into the Olympics has not been successful, but since 1994 the Commonwealth Games have included various demonstration sports for what they patronisingly refer to as 'Elite Athletes with a Disability'. Since the Commonwealth Games in Manchester during 2002 these events have had full medal status (Smith and Thomas 2005) – something of which the founders of CIAD would be proud.

Seoul, South Korea 1988

The Seoul Paralympics of 1988 were a watershed in the history of the Paralympic Movement. For the first time, Paralympic athletes were given the opportunity to compete using the best sporting facilities that the world had to offer. These Games started the transformation from a participation-based model of sport for the disabled to the high-performance model that exists today. Medals were not as plentiful as they had been in the last two Paralympiads, thus increasing their value to the winner (though there were some events and classes that still held strong to the participation ethos of the Games) and starting the transformation to where a Paralympic Champion should be as highly prized as an Olympic Champion.

Organisation of the Paralympics was taken to heart by the Koreans, and the Seoul Paralympic Organising Committee (SPOC) had a positive relationship with the organisers of the Olympic Games. One problem that faced the SPOC was that it was unsure how best to run the Paralympics. This lack of knowledge was ultimately of benefit to the Paralympic Movement, since the organisers staged the Games following the same format that had been used at the Olympics:

> It is the first time that the Olympics and the Paralympic Organizing Committees are making an integrated and co-ordinated effort in order for human resources and sport installations to be fully utilized.
>
> (Park 1987: 501)

The village for the Paralympics was a short distance from the Olympic Stadium, and consisted of ten purpose-built apartment buildings which housed everyone involved with the Games. While this established a Paralympic 'family' environment, there were issues with the infrastructure. Elevators in the tower blocks could only handle two wheelchairs at a time, and as a result those athletes who were ambulant were housed on the upper floors of the tower blocks and required to climb fifteen floors to and from the rooms. Some of the buildings had long ramps down the side to allow wheelchair athletes to descend, which, though dangerous, were a source of amusement to the non-risk-adverse in the wheelchair fraternity who would race each other down the ramps in a side-by-side fashion on adjoining buildings.

To mark the push to high-profile sport through creditable events at the Paralympic Games, 156 events largely involving athletes with a severe disability had to be cancelled because there were fewer than three athletes in each field. This move created a great deal of tension between the ICC and the nations. It is a concern that still exists today (Jones and Howe 2005; Howe and Jones 2006), in the sense that high-performance sport is not only premised upon the training regime that is involved with regard to a certain event, but also on the number of individuals that are internationally willing to undergo a similar regime to create a viable competition. The ICC insisted the move would solidify its serious intent to run an elite sporting event but the IOSDs (which were founded on a participation platform) were by and large disappointed.

The opening ceremony on 15 October was held in the Olympic stadium and was the same as that at the Olympics, only the processing athletes had impairments. It was an event that was held in front of a capacity crowd of 75 000, and each the athletes was every bit an Olympian. The Movement had gathered pace after 1984, and sixty-one countries and a record number of 3053 athletes were involved. For the first time a Paralympic flag flew over the stadium, adapting the internationally recognisable Olympic rings using five *Tae-Geuk*, which is a traditional Korean decorative motif (see Figure 2.1), after the Games were declared open by Mr Roh Tae-Woo, President of the Republic of Korea.

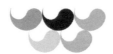

Figure 2.1 Paralympic logo 1988–1993. © International Paralympic Committee.

Barcelona 1992

Continuing the progress toward the high-performance model of sport that was started in Seoul four years earlier, Barcelona was the first Games where the IPC had influence. Following a meeting held with the IOSDs, the nations and the ICC, the International Paralympic Committee (IPC) was established in 1989 and Canadian Dr Robert Steadward became its first President. In light of these developments, the organising committee for the Olympic Games felt that it needed to police the quality of the Paralympics. In part, it was concerned the that vast number of different classes and small number of competitors within each class would detract from the Paralympics as a viable sporting spectacle. The organising committee established strict regulations, such as the need for there to be six athletes from at least four different countries who had performed at or above the entry standard for the event to be viable at the Games. This was helped by the move to create an integrated functional classification system within the sport of swimming in 1989, which ultimately made the sport less likely to cancel events and did reduce the number of competitors (Vanlande-wijck and Chappel 1996; Daly and Vanlandewijck 1999; Dummer 1999). Along with coaches and administrators, 3000 athletes were housed in the village which had been used during the Olympic Games, as it was largely accessible throughout. Funding for the Games was limited by the Olympic organisers, but the Spanish National Organisation for the Blind (ONCE) established a lottery, the profits of which were used to facilitate the high-quality Games.

Taking a page out of the Seoul organising committee's handbook, the opening ceremony was again a repeat of the one used at the Olympics. A capacity crowd of 65000 spectators attended, and it was watched by millions of television viewers. There were teams from ninety-four nations, and the strong show of support from the Olympic Movement was embodied by the presence of Spain' s President of the International Olympic Committee (IOC), Juan Antonio Samaranch. In all, over the fifteen days of competition more than one-and-a-half million spectators attended the event, in part because admission to all events other than the opening and closing ceremonies was free. There were 431 gold medals won among over 3000 athletes, highlighting that the push toward the elite model of sport had been successfully undertaken. In the nearby city of Madrid, seventy-three nations competed in the Games for athletes with intellectual disabilities. In four years' time this disability group would have a mixed reception as it officially joined the Paralympic Movement in Atlanta in 1996.

As the Movement continued to gain momentum, the IOC questioned the close resemblance between IPC logo and their own and as a result threatened to

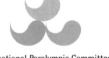

International Paralympic Committee

Figure 2.2   Paralympic logo 1994–2002. © International Paralympic Committee.

break ties with the IPC if the logo was not changed (Mason 2002). The move to a new logo was not to the liking of many within the Paralympic Movement, but there was a willingness in the IPC corridors of power to adopt the logo to please the IOC (Steadward 2000). From 1994 until 2003 the logo was an adaptation of the Tae-Geuk concept adopted in Seoul, and was often accompanied by the motto 'Mind, Body and Spirit' (see Figure 2.2).

Atlanta 1996

A new IOSD, the International Sports Federation for Persons with Intellectual Disability (INAS-FID), was welcomed to the Movement at the Atlanta Paralympics. Many athletes from the more established disability groups were concerned that the inclusion of this federation's athletes would undermine the success of the Paralympic Movement, which was already having difficulty distinguishing itself from the Special Olympics – which at that time had a very participation-driven focus. Some commentators have argued that there is a pecking order for the different disability groups (Sherrill and Williams 1996) in terms of who has a viable claim to be involved in disability sport and who is considered to be 'normal' within this abnormal world. My observations and notes taken at the Atlanta Games suggest that athletes with intellectual disability were at the bottom of the hierarchy, since many athletes felt that the able bodies of this impairment group meant quite simply that they should not be eligible for the Paralympic Games. After all, there are many professional sportsmen who have questionable intelligence, but they are allowed to compete with the best able-bodied athletes.

Through cooperation with the local organising committee, the IPC again made great strides in its attempt to guarantee the high quality of performances at the Games. Developing a system that ensured more dynamic growth and improvement within each sport event, the IPC attempted to allow only viable events onto the final competition programme. This system was based on the three key components of quality, quantity and universality. In essence, the system was developed to eliminate events that were not attracting a high-quality field of competitors. On the back of this streamlining of the programme, the organisers were able to include more nations by offering financial assistance to some National Paralympic Committees from the 'developing' world. This initiative was such a success that there were 121 nations present in Atlanta, with almost 3200 athletes involved in twenty sports; three – wheelchair rugby (made famous to non-Paralympic audiences in the documentary *Murderball*), sailing and racquetball – were held as demonstrations.

Atlanta was not a success in terms of attendance. While almost 400000 people attended the Games, this was well down on the figures from Barcelona. One of the main reasons for this was that tickets were *sold* in Atlanta, as the organisers felt that no one would go to an event if it were free – reflecting cultural differences between the Southern United States and the heart of Catalonia. The opening and closing ceremonies were well attended, but were not sell-outs. Paralympic merchandise was available in a wide variety of outlets around the city, and for the first time the Games attracted a worldwide sponsor in the form of Coca-Cola®. The Atlanta Paralympic organisers became the first in the Movement's history to develop a licensing programme whereby manufacturers could, for a price, be seen to be officially associated with the Paralympic Games (BBC 1994). There were also over 2000 media accreditations, highlighting the growing interest in the Movement.

The educational imperative of the IPC came to the fore during the Games. A Paralympic Congress was organised several days prior to the competition, the theme of which was the political and economic empowerment of people with disabilities, as well as more general global issues in sport for the disabled. A cultural pyramid existed at the Games which exhibited work from disabled artists and was designed to allow viewers to draw similarities between excellence in the creative endeavour of art and the physical prowess of sport.

Sydney 2000

Further symmetry was brought to the relationship between the Olympic and Paralympic Movements at the Games in Sydney. For the first time, the core services of the Paralympic Games were dealt with by the same people who organised the Olympics. So determined were they that this would take place, the Australians marketed the Olympics and Paralympics as the 'Sixty Day Sporting Festival' (Cashman 2006). The Paralympics used the same village as the Olympics, with the same high-quality catering, medical care and entertainment venues. This was a great improvement over Atlanta, where the rooms were seldom cleaned (to the point that they were unhygienic) and the food was of poor quality and served up in hothouse conditions. Issues relating to transport, tickets for events and the technology required to host the Games were passed on with the ease of a torch relay from the Olympics to the Paralympics.

A record number of countries (123, including the highly publicised attendance of East Timor) participated in the XI Paralympic Games. The Paralympic Village housed almost 7000 people, including 3824 athletes who fought for 550 sets of medals. The media attention surrounding the Games was again intense, with 2300 members of the media gaining accreditation. With advances in technology the Games were able to be webcast[7] for the first time through a sponsorship deal through WeMedia, who agreed to videostream 100 hours of competition on the Internet. Over 100 countries were able to log in to the webcast, and there were reportedly 300 million hits on the Games' official website over the fortnight. Interest in the Games was not, however, all in cyberspace. Sydney attracted 1.2 million paying spectators – over three times as Atlanta four years earlier, and almost as many as Barcelona, where admittance was free (Cashman 2006).

This social history is important in helping those unfamiliar with the Paralympic Movement to make sense of its philosophy. The roots of Paralympism are embedded in the history of both the rehabilitative and the participatory models highlighted above, but it is now a production of the marketing during the high-performance era in which we currently exist.

Roots of Paralympism

Paralympism is an ideology celebrated by the IPC that has been developed in an attempt to establish a universal ethos that extends beyond the Paralympic Games, in much the same manner that Olympism has transcended the more established Olympic Games. Some scholars working within the field of sport for the disabled have argued that a philosophy of Paralympism is not needed since Olympism is appropriate for the Paralympic Movement (Wolff *et al.*, in press). Clearly there are examples of harmony between Paralympism and Olympism. The motto of the Barcelona '92 IXth Paralympic Games 'Sport without limits', resonates with Olympism.

The International Olympic Committee's definition is believed by some to reflect the centrality of Coubertin's vision. The fundamental principles of the Olympic Movement, enshrined in the *Olympic Charter* (International Olympic Committee 2004: 9), suggest that

> Olympism is a philosophy of life, exalting and combining in a balanced whole the qualities of body, will and mind. Blending sport with culture and education, Olympism seeks to create a way of life based on the joy of effort, the educational value of good example and respect for universal fundamental ethical principles.

and further that

> The goal of Olympism is to place sport at the service of the harmonious development of man, with a view to promoting a peaceful society concerned with the preservation of human dignity.

Taking this at face value, 'the expression "Paralympism" appears to be somewhat superfluous, pleonastic; "Olympism" is sufficient … it says it all' (Landry 1995: 5). In fact, during the 1956 Olympic Games 'the International Olympic Committee awarded the Fearnley Cup to the organisers of the International Stoke Mandeville Games [the antecedent of the Paralympics] for "outstanding achievement in the service of Olympic ideals"' (Goodman 1986: 157). Yet for those concerned with cultural political issues surrounding sport for the disabled to limit the Paralympic practice community (see Howe and Jones 2006) to an ideology that has not been specifically created for them goes against the grain of the cultural evolution of the Movement.

According to Parry (2004: 1), 'Olympism is a social philosophy which emphasises the role of sport in world development, international understanding, peaceful co-existence, and social and moral education'. As a result, compliance with it in practice can add virtue to the Paralympic Movement. However, since the Paralympic Movement has a distinctive cultural history and resulting habitus to match, the need to establish an understanding of Paralympism is paramount. There are those who advocate simply the use of Olympism (Wolff *et al.* in press) as a sign of the growing harmony between the Olympic and Paralympic Movements because discrimination of individuals regardless of ability is against the principle tenants of Olympism. In practice, however, both the Olympic and Paralympic Games exclude the (dis)abled or, to put it another way, 'those who can't'. Yes, Olympism may be an inclusive ideology (Wolff *et al.* in press), but the practice of high-performance sport is not (Howe and Jones 2006).

The Paralympic Movement has raised public consciousness, both transnationally as well as trans-culturally, with respect to the philosophical concept and meaning of *human* performance (Howe and Jones 2006). As such, it has allowed for the debate regarding Western sporting practice (ethos) and places virtue at the feet those who achieve excellence in measurable sporting terms (Landry 1995). In this respect, the achievements of Paralympians will never achieve the same status as those of Olympians.

Almost two decades ago Labanowich (1988) argued for the integration of the Paralympic Games into the Olympics, based upon the number of countries and athletes contesting various sports within the Paralympic Games. While there may be some validity in this move, the essence of Paralympism might have been lost. To start Coubertin in *The Fundamentals of the Philosophy of the Modern Olympics* (1956 [1935]: 53), highlights the degree to which physical culture may be used as a vehicle to achieve sporting excellence when he states:

> For a hundred men to take part in physical education, you must have fifty who go in for sport. For fifty to go in for sport, you must have twenty to specialise, you must have five who are capable of remarkable physical feats.

This is not a situation that is commonplace in Paralympic sport. There is exceedingly stiff competition to get into certain events at the Paralympic Games, notably class T54[8] – the most 'able' of wheelchair racers, where selection is tough (if not tougher) than for the Olympic Games – but technology is a factor here. It is clear, from data collected in the context of Paralympic Athletics, that it is easier across the board to be selected for the Paralympic than for the Olympic Games. This is the case because many of the classes of impaired athletes struggle to get enough competitors to reach the qualifying standards for the Paralympic Games. To my knowledge, this has never been the case at the Olympics.

The Paralympic Movement as a whole does not create a sporting aristocracy, as Coubertin believed the Olympics did, but it has created its own rituals, some of which are a direct parroting of those used by the Olympic Movement. For example, the opening and closing ceremonies, since 1988, have been replicated to a high degree at the Paralympics, assuring a full house on opening and closing nights. The establishment of the dictum 'empower, inspire and achieve' at the heart Paralympism is distinct from the Olympic motto. In a sense, the Paralympic Games cannot follow Coubertin's vision of the cycle of Olympiad to provide the youth of any moment in time with the opportunity to compete in an international context. By stating 'The Springtime of human life is found in the young adult who may be compared to a superb machine up and ready to enter, into full activity' (Coubertin 1956 [1935]: 53–54), Coubertin believed that the Olympics were an ideal environment for fostering the youth (his own strong affinity with the Fascist regime in Germany during the 1930s aside). Many athletes who compete in the Paralympic Games of the past and today are 'eligible' as a result of a traumatic occurrence in life which clearly has no fixed time in the development of the individual. Rehabilitation in a sense can be about creating another individual, or a re-birth (Seymour 1998). In other words, Paralympians are generally older than Olympians, and rehabilitation continues to be a feature of contemporary sport for the disabled.

While the 1896 Athens Games took place under the shadow of a war in nearby Crete (MacAloon 1981), the first international sporting event for the disabled (at least the one seen as the first event in terms of Paralympic history) took place in Stoke Mandeville on the day of the opening ceremony for the 1948 London Games. The athletes were all ex-service personnel – fourteen men and two women casualties of the war. These individuals were the product of Guttmann's rehabilitative medicine. From those early days there has been a transformation in the Paralympic Movement from a model of participation to one of high performance sport (see Howe 2004a; Jones and Howe 2005).

While the International Paralympic Committee has distanced itself from any explicit discussion of Paralympism, relying instead on the dictum *Empower, Inspire, Achieve*, the vision of the Movement is 'To Enable Paralympic Athletes to Achieve Sporting Excellence and Inspire and Excite the World'. The only official statement of Paralympism comes from the Asian Paralympic Committee,[9] which clearly is enamoured with Olympism.

> Paralympism is a philosophy of life which embraces the mind, body and spirit. By combining sport with education, Paralympism aims to nurture a way of life for persons with a disability based on effort, good example and respect for ethics. The ideals of Paralympism encompass both the promotion and development of 'Sport For All' and 'Elite Sports'. Although each has differing philosophy, fundamental goals and objectives, they complement each other and stress lifelong education and experience, values, traditions and fair play, towards attaining long term individual, social, cultural and economic goals.

The Paralympic Movement, like that of the Olympics, 'benefited from the benign myths of origin rooted in reverential attitudes toward the personal qualities of their respective founding fathers and the salvational doctrine they created' (Hoberman 1995: 3). Guttmann would anger at athletes flexing their muscles as individuals and attempting to suggest a different direction for the

Stoke Mandeville Games. An informant – an athlete who competed internationally in sport for the disabled events in the 1960s and 70s – stated:

> Guttmann was in many respects a great man. By the time I had come into sport he was perceived as an emperor. His word was law. There were a number of occasions at major events when he blew his top. This often occurred when athletes had suggested things might be organised differently for the next event. He did not like change unless he initiated it. Guttmann was an exceedingly strong character.

In many respects the fledgling Paralympic Movement that Guttmann ruled over is not dissimilar to the world of corruption, brought on by a distinct lack of surveillance – in part by the myth associated with Olympism (that it actually existed), how involvement with the IOC meant material reward, and a 'long history of extreme right-wing personalities and attitudes within the IOC' – uncovered in the *Lord of the Rings* (see Hoberman 1995: 6).

The truth behind the Olympic Movement is that the chivalric tendencies of the Movement, the knightly ethos of officials and athletes alike, 'was the precise negation of socialist rationality, solidarity, and the improvement of ordinary life for the greatest number' (Hoberman 1995: 19). While de Coubertin created 'The Myth of the War experience' (Hoberman 1995: 20) – the simple idea of military heroism – many Paralympians, at least in the early days, lived it though they were often treated as 'less than men'. Unlike de Coubertin's original version of the idealised male action figure, the 'débrouillard', the dynamic 'go-getter' type (Hoberman 1995: 22), Paralympians were broadly seen as charity cases. As such, it is not surprising that the Paralympic Games was seen as detrimental for the broader Disabled Persons Movement. Guttmann best summed this up in 1976 when he scored an own goal in his classic pronouncement, '*Mens sana in corpore sano* (Healthy mind in healthy body) should read *Mens sana in corpore sano et invalido!* (Healthy mind in healthy body and infirm [weak or feeble] body)' (Guttmann 1976: 13). This statement highlights what the Paralympic Movement is in part about – providing high-performance sporting opportunities for less than able bodies. Ultimately Paralympism, as personified in the dictum *Empower, Inspire, Achieve*, is a goal worth pursuing, but, given the direction the Paralympic Movement is heading, it will be difficult to attain.

Summary

The origin and growth of the Paralympic Movement from the 'first International Games for the Disabled in Rome' (DePauw and Gavron 1995: 37) in 1960 has been combined with a change of emphasis in the nature of international sport for the disabled. The original Games were 'influenced by the medical establishment, with disability and rehabilitation' (Steadward 1996: 28). However, the evolution of the sport for the disabled movement has led to the formation of a new set of ideals for the Paralympic Movement. Participation was the hallmark of the early international event, but by 1972 officials were keen to codify the practice of sport for the disabled. This act was the catalyst for a slow progression to a high-performance Paralympic Games. A major step in this evolution occurred as a result of the establishment of the International Paralympic Committee (IPC) in Düsseldorf on 21 September 1989. The new movement was designed to promote sport for the disabled – 'sport for sport's sake and competition for competition's sake' (DePauw and Gavron 1995: 223). This shift from rehabilitation to participation and then finally to achievement sport has come at a price. 'Body, Mind and Spirit' was in a sense an unsuitable motto for the Movement, since it is in fact the bodies of impaired athletes that often negatively segregate them from the mainstream. These and other debates will be fleshed out later in the monograph.

3 Paralympic 'lived history'

Reflections of a participant observer

With the establishment of the Stoke Mandeville Games, the antecedent of the Paralympic Games, participation was considered the most important part of provision in sport for the disabled. The rehabilitative nature of sport for the disabled will always be in the background, as athletes who suffer traumatic injury will need rehabilitation before being able to participate in sport. Likewise, it takes athletes a while to become accomplished enough as participants in order become involved in high-performance sporting practice, the current pinnacle of which is the Paralympic Games.

In a sense, my entry into the field was at the nexus between the eras of participation and high performance. Athletes who trained and prepared for the high-performance sport in the mid-1980s were the new breed of Paralympians that dominates in the mass sporting spectacles that the Movement is showcased through two decades later. No longer are athletes encouraged or increasingly able to compete at the international level in two distinct sports, since the standards of performances and the number of athletes competing for the limited number of places available on teams has meant vastly increased competition for places. During the World Championships of the summer of 1986, many of the athletes and coaches were from the participation culture era of sport for the disabled – the 'old guard' – and the tensions with athletes with a high-performance agenda were clear to see. The training regimes of less than a quarter of the athletes when I first got involved in sport for the disabled were, from observation, high performance. Currently, I would estimate four of every five athletes are training to an elite level.

The 1984 Paralympic Games marked the end of an era that had advocated the importance of sports participation in the lives of impaired individuals. Problems with organising the Games meant that they were held in two different countries. Athletes from ISOD, CP-ISRA and IBSA all competed in events held in New York, where as ISMWSF athletes held their part of the Paralympic Games at Stoke Mandeville Hospital near Aylesbury in the United Kingdom. In spite of the geographical dichotomy, this was a watershed moment for the Paralympic Movement because, during the Los Angeles Olympics of the same year, two wheelchair races were held in the athletics programme – a 1500 m event for men and an 800 m event for women. In the Winter Olympics in Sarajevo of the same year, skiing events for the disabled were held for the first time. These high-profile demonstrations gave the embryonic Paralympic Movement a great deal of positive exposure, but, perhaps more importantly, facilitated a change in attitude among young people with disabilities – that high-performance sport was acceptable for impaired athletes. Many of these athletes had been training seriously, driven to succeed by the achievements of many able-bodied heroes. The realisation that impaired athletes could do the same created a ground swell of interest in the opportunities for elite athletes with a disability.

Early exposure on the able-bodied sporting stage was reserved for wheelchair users, which is not particularly surprising because the development of organised sport for the disabled (at least as it pertains to the Paralympic Movement) started with early development of sporting programmes, following the Second World War at Stoke Mandeville Hospital, where the ISMWSF has its roots (see Chapter 2). The negative side of this increased exposure for ISMWSF athletes was that it could be seen to be the trigger for a process of marginalisation of other disabled groups within the Paralympic Movement (see Chapter 8). Sherrill and Williams (1996) have suggested that there is an order of importance within athletes of various impairment groups, with ISMWSF competitors being top of the tree, followed by the amputee and the blind, while bringing up the rear are those who are part of the CP-ISRA. The research was conducted before the INAS-FID was part of the Paralympic family, but it can be assumed that this group of athletes would now have a similar standing to athletes with cerebral palsy. INAS-FID athletes have intellectual impairments and there have been implicit assumptions since I became involved in Paralympic athletics that many cerebral palsy are also intellectually disabled. Athletes who use wheelchairs or prosthetic limbs most often acquire their impairments from a trauma that occurs after birth – in other words, they were socialised as normal individuals and, but for fate, would not be in the disabled world. Both people with intellectual disability and those with cerebral palsy often either have trouble with communication or were socialised in a way that was a result of their impairment. The impairment is disabling often as a result of time spent in segregated educational environments. As such, the act of socialisation may be distinctive from that in athletes who have normal mental functioning but have become impaired through a life experience. As Cashman (2006: 247) recently commented, '[t]he "hierarchy of acceptability" is another problem faced by Paralympic organisers in that some athlete categories featured more prominently than others because they are more easily understood by the non-disabled majority who watch Paralympic telecasts'.

In some respects it was a blessing when I first became aware of the stigma (see Goffman 1963) associated with being an athlete with cerebral palsy. My initial experience with fellow CP-ISRA athletes left me feeling rather ill at ease, simply because I did not have anything in common with the majority of them other than my impairment. By and large, they were more interested in drinking alcohol and partying than they were in preparing for competition at both training camps and during competition – and while I have nothing against the drinking of alcohol, it does have its time and place. If the athletes who competed for the ISMWSF, the ISOD and the IBSA were looking down on those who competed for the CP-ISRA, I felt that rather than it being linked to how the individual impairment was acquired it was more about the socialisation into sport. Was an athlete there to participate or to perform? I shared a desire with many others of the so-called 'new breed' of Paralympians in the mid-1980s simply to compete to the best of my ability, but importantly to train as hard as elite able-bodied athletes in order to achieve success.

It appears that the stigma of being a CP-ISRA performer rather than a participant took some time to remove. The realisation on the part of athletes from other IOSDs that not all members of the CP-ISRA are cut from the same participatory cloth took time, as one high-profile wheelchair athlete commented during the 1992 Barcelona Paralympic Games:

> Many of the CP athletes I have nothing in common with. The ones in [wheel]chairs don't seem to train with the same intensity that we do and many of the ambulant ones simply don't look like they train at all. Overweight and lazy – here for a holiday. As I get to know more of them I can see that there are some highly trained members of the squad that have CP but so many of them don't appear to be here for the same reasons as us.

The professionalism of the approach to training became a key marker that separated many of the competitors in the various federations in the mid-1980s. By the time of the 1992 Paralympic Games, there was still a residual participation ethos within the Paralympic Movement. Many of the paternalistic members of IOSDs, who believed in the participation model of sport for the disabled, had been sidelined, but a number were still in positions of influence. By the time of the Games in Athens in 2004 the ethos of high performance was all that there was room for, as the IPC was pressurised after signing an agreement with the IOC (IPC 2003a) to limit the size of Paralympic Games to 4000 competitors. However, in the mid-1980s the there was a good deal of tension between those who advocated the participation model of sport for the disabled and those who were eager that high performance (based on the model of the Olympic Games) was the way forward.

Seoul 1988

In the autumn of 1988, directly following the Olympic Games in Seoul, the hosts agreed to stage the Paralympic Games. This was a coming of age for the Paralympic Movement because, with limited experience in organising multi-disability sporting festivals, the organisers did the only thing they knew how to do – ran the Paralympics on the same model as the Olympics. This is, of course, a format that has, with mixed degrees of success, been adopted by all host nations since. It was a watershed simply because the organisers in Korea felt that Paralympians needed to be treated with the same respect as Olympians. There were, of course, hiccups in the running of the Games. For example, the elevators in the Paralympic village could only carry two wheelchair users at a time, and this meant that all ambulant athletes at least were on the sixth floor of the tower blocks and were required to use the stairs, or to wait an hour for a lift. This minor inconvenience allowed the Paralympians to appear to be treated in a similar fashion to the Olympians.

There was a real sense around the village that the Movement was coming of age. Many of the participants from the trip to Belgium two years earlier were not selected for the team. The build-up to the Seoul Games facilitated my first detailed observations of other impairment groups. The teams had representatives from the ISMWSF, the IBSA and the ISOD as well as the CP-ISRA, and this facilitated an opportunity to see first-hand how these groups interacted. Athletes from the ISMWSF and the wheelchair users from the CP-ISRA were housed in the lower extremities of the tower blocks that the teams occupied because of their need to have better access to the lifts. Because of the lack of independence experienced by some of the CP athletes, particularly classes 1 and 2, they were often not invited to socialise and were *de facto* excluded from the social environment of the ISMWSF athletes. Some of this may have been a result of the fact that many members of the more severely impaired cerebral palsy classes find it difficult to communicate orally, so striking up a conversation takes an effort on the behalf of both parties. It may have been lack of opportunity for conversation, or it may have been that athletes with CP were not perceived as being serious athletes. Each group of athletes has a distinctive understanding of their impairment and the various classes of competitors that make up the group. A lack of understanding of other groups' impairment may sometimes lead to a situation where some feel marginalised by the lack of understanding and awareness of others.

The manner in which impairment groups relate to one another is of course not particular to sport for the disabled or the disability communitas; rather, it is a universal social condition. While people who have impairments rebel against the process that facilitates them being 'othered' by society at large (Oliver 1996; Tisdall 2003), this does not mean that within the disabled sporting communitas the same process does not occur. It would be wrong to assume that all sports people with impairments share such a strong bond that the stigmatising that occurs throughout society does not occur within sport for the disabled. The political environment surrounding the transformation from participant- to performance-mode of sporting practice meant that those with vested interests were keen to shape the Paralympic Movement to meet their needs. Effectively, each group of athletes, by excluding, teasing and targeting others without getting to know them, caused these groups to seldom socialise together. On the macro level, the federations, largely staffed by volunteers who were able-bodied, had also established their own hierarchy of importance, which meant that when the IPC was formed in 1989 officials with the old ISMWSF gained the most influential positions.

No doubt the political manoeuvring required to achieve these positions was going on before and during the Games in Seoul, but since it would be another eight years until I was able to access the decision-making structures of the Movement (albeit as a lowly representative of the athletes on the International Paralympic Committee Athletics Committee), observations during these Games were restricted to interactions with the athletes and their environment. On the whole, there was a slightly more professional approach by athletes to the Games in Seoul. No longer was it considered acceptable for athletes to consume alcohol in the village, and all members of the Canadian delegation were asked to sign a statement that they would abide by certain rules or be sent home at their own expense. In discussion with fellow athletes from other Western nations, it became clear that they were required to do the same. Whether the host nation did the same was unclear, but they had a strong, well-disciplined team that performed very well across the board.

It might be worth noting here that the Korean people came out in large numbers to support their athletes and welcome those from around the world. At the flagship venues of the athletics track in the Olympic stadium, the swimming pool and the basketball stadium, spectators attended in their thousands. The Olympic stadium was at least 25 per cent full for my heats (the biggest crowd I had run in front of until then), and athletes were mobbed by enthusiastic schoolchildren on the concourses around the Olympic venues. After my 800 m final I was feeling rather dejected, having been placed seventh, and a group of us were walking back to catch the bus for the village when we were surrounded by over a hundred schoolchildren who were eager to obtain our autographs. We stood there and signed our autographs for almost an hour as other school groups joined the frenzy. This attention made us forget our 'bad' performances of the day. While on reflection the kids were no doubt sent out by their schools on projects that encouraged them to collect our autographs, this type of reception made us all feel good about ourselves. It certainly engrained in us the meaning of representing our various countries; whether those school projects served a long-term educational purpose is another matter.

What has been the legacy of the Seoul Paralympic Games? Clearly the Korean team was bigger than any other they have sent to subsequent Games, but what appears to be of greater importance is how people with impairments are treated within Korean society at large. When athletes grew bored of the refectory food available in the village, they would take a taxi to the central business district – an area that appeared to be at the heart of Western consumerism, where all the products shipped to the West were copied and sold at significantly reduced prices. Stalls in the streets were selling all sorts of imitation designer goods, as well as cheaply tailored suits where quality matched the price. This area was accessed by taxi from the village, and the drivers seemed to be at ease with taking passengers who were in wheelchairs (especially if the wheels could easily be removed from the chair) – something that even today, in the West, can be problematic from time to time.

None of the restaurants in this part of Seoul were wheelchair-accessible, and on more than one occasion we had to lift athletes up a large narrow staircase so that they could have share the dining splendour that was Pizza Hut. No doubt the centres of cities like Seoul are more accessible now than they were in the late 1980s, as are cities like London and New York in the West. Clearly access issues were also high on the agenda of pioneers in the field of disability studies who were, at least initially, working in the Western context. Mike Oliver, in his landmark text *The Politics of Disablement* (1990), captured the mood of the period by including a photograph of a man in a wheelchair at the foot of a flight of stairs outside a polling station.

Issues of access were key to the success of the Seoul Paralympics. While the built environment was not ideal as trips around the city suggested, a desire to compensate for the lack of accessible infrastructure and an openness of attitude appeared to be at the heart of the Games organising committee. If issues of access had been completely addressed by the Games organising committee, then the establishment of the IPC a year after Seoul might have taken a different focus. As it was, the IPC assumed the role of organising the Paralympic Games (both winter and summer) as its primary mandate. Choosing this role obviously gave the IPC the sort of influential position it desired without the need to con-sider the seemingly more tedious issues of grass-roots development of athletes, which became the responsibility of the IOSDs. It was a structural shift of polit-ical significance, because in a single meeting the IPC was empowered and IOSDs and the athletes were disempowered. Quite simply, it placed the IPC at the centre of the Paralympic Movement.

Establishment of the IPC

In 1982, as international sport for the disabled was receiving more support, particularly in the West, the IOSDs formed a new umbrella organisation named the International Coordinating Committee of the World Sports Organisations (ICC). The two primary aims of this organisation were to organise sport for the disabled internationally, and to negotiate with the IOC on behalf of athletes with a disability. This organisation provided an opportunity for nations and the IOSDs to attempt to secure a better future for athletes with a disability. On 14 March 1987, in Arnham, the Netherlands, during a seminar run by the ICC, it was decided that a new inclusive organisation would be formed which would have representatives from all nations that ran sport for the disabled programmes as well as the IOSDs (DePauw and Gavron 1995: 44). Importantly, athletes were to have a voice in issues of governance at the international level.

Bathing in the relative success of the Paralympic Games in Seoul, the ICC and the *ad hoc* committee charged with steering an athlete-centred, national representative organisation announced the establishment of the IPC in Düssel-dorf, Germany, on 21 and 22 September 1989. At these meetings, officers were elected and the governance structure (including a draft constitution) was adopted. The first stage was for the IPC to streamline the organisation of inter-national sport (DePauw and Gavron 2005) and, importantly, to establish close links with the IOC. The transition between the ICC and the IPC went smoothly at the completion of the 1992 Paralympic Games in Barcelona. Since taking over the mantle of power from the ICC, the IPC has gone to great lengths to stress that it is an athlete-centred organisation. There has been a desire for the publicity rhetoric to reflect that the IPC is an athlete-centred organisation with the best interest of the athletes at heart.

The reality of the situation is somewhat less clear. Athletes are centre-stage and an important part of what the IPC does – after all, it is the IPC's mandate to run the Paralympic Games, and athletes are required in order for the show to go on. However the structure of the organisation suggests that the presence of athletes is of little or no importance to the successful running of the administrative side of the organisation.[1] It is clear from this structure that the athletes' committee is not centre-stage, and there is no provision for the active recruitment of former Paralympians to positions of influence (though the second President is a former athlete). If the organisation had been established to facilitate opportunities for women, for example, there would most certainly be an active policy to recruit them into positions of power.

Liaising with the IOC on the relationship between it and the IPC has given the President of the IPC a considerable amount of influence. As the relationship between the IPC and the IOC has become closer (IPC 2001, 2003b), the initial assumption that the IPC would be distinct from the IOC in terms of being a more athlete-focused organisation is possibly as naive as the view that the ideology that helped to found the Olympic Movement still has salience for the IOC political members today. This not to suggest that Olympism is of no value, but rather that the majority of the political figures in the Movement simply pay lip service to this ideology as a result of the importance of attracting multinational corporate sponsorship.

Barcelona 1992

This was the last Games before the IPC assumed power over the organisation, though many of the officials who were involved with the ICC would become key figures in the new power brokerage of disabled sport. As an event for the athletes, coaches and support staff, the 1992 Games were a huge success. Much like Seoul four years earlier, there was considerable interest from the local communitas. The organisers had decided that the event should be an educational opportunity for the people of Spain, and as a result did not charge admission to competition venues. In the finals for track and field events, the stadium was full. Unlike Seoul, where most of the observers were there apparently as part of school trips, the stadium seemed to be full of citizens of Barcelona from all walks of life. The opening and closing ceremonies at the Games were a huge spectacle and were the only events for which tickets were required – in part because the organising committee used the same performances that the Olympic had a month earlier, and many of the locals had been unable to attend these events live. This mix created an electric atmosphere that was only enhanced by the hot, humid conditions. Athletes had been warned by their various NPCs of the climatic conditions with which they would be confronted; the onus four years previously had been on the athletes to ascertain the type of climatic conditions they would be confronted with in Seoul. Climatically both venues were similar, though the heavy pollution that seemed to envelop the city of Seoul (factories were closed during the Olympics but back in full production for the Paralympic Games) was not present in Barcelona.

The Paralympic village, situated on the Mediterranean, was well organised and accessible, and the athletes were housed in apartment blocks where there was social space as well as accommodation, which was organised two athletes per room. As an accessible site it was much better than Seoul, with the apartment blocks only three or four stories tall, and more elevators. One of the big adjustments that was successfully made to the site were two large ramps, one in and one out of the dining hall which was in the centre of the village. For the first time there was also provision for entertainment in the village, such as bowling alleys and a cinema, which helped to pass the time between training and the culmination of competition. The Games were so successfully run that one of the chief organisers, Xavier Gonzalez, went on to be chief organiser of both the Atlanta 1996 and the Sydney 2000 Games before taking up a full-time post as Chief Executive Officer with the IPC just prior to the Athens 2004 Paralympic Games.

In terms of transportation to and from the main competition venues, the organisation of the Spanish hosts could not be questioned, and the enthusiasm for the Games by the local population meant that wherever athletes ventured out of the village or venues they were well treated. Even if the city of Barcelona was not as accessible as some athletes would have liked, the willingness to accommodate all forms of mobility impairment eased issues that were problematic in the built environment. A sign of the professionalism in the Paralympic Movement was that Barcelona marked the first occasion where drug-testing took place. No doubt the public outcry following Ben Johnson's positive test in Seoul meant that if the Paralympic Movement was going to follow the lead of the IOC it needed to assure the public that star performers were clean. This is, of course, a sad sign of the times – when a sports organisation gains enough respectability that some athletes want to cheat to win. It would be another eight years before I became aware of the extent to which the use of performance-enhancing drugs was a problem.

It was in Barcelona that I also became aware that the coaching provision, at least within the Canadian team, was becoming more professional. The whole squad was better prepared, and there was a professional attitude within the team. In athletics, however, there were a couple of incidents that soured my enjoyment, in part because they illustrated how winning was all that really mattered. I am aware that the reader might feel there is a contradiction here. Winning is important in sport, and I always trained to do just that; however, I believe that certain ethics need to be adhered to in order maintain fair play (Loland 2002).

One of the Canadian team, a class T38 sprinter (the most minimally impaired class of cerebral palsy athlete eligible to compete), who had acquired CP through a head trauma, won three gold medals at the Games. However, during the lap of honour following his final race, the athlete was involved in a fight with a competitor from another country. He was subsequently sent home by the Canadian team early in an attempt to diffuse the situation. To my knowledge he was not banned from competing for Canada for any period of time, and was certainly a member of the team that attended the IPC Athletics World Championships in Berlin during the summer of 1994.

One of the reasons given for not suspending the athlete was that his cerebral palsy was a result of a head injury. There are a number of issues here that are relevant to the debates relating to classification that are on going within the Paralympic Movement (see Chapter 4). In my view, regardless of whether the individual had in the past suffered a head injury, the athlete should not have become involved in any form of physical misbehaviour. The unofficial response to this incident was that the unacceptable behaviour could have been the product of a head injury. Some within the Canadian contingent, myself included, were ill at ease about how the situation was handled, thinking that a ban might have been more appropriate as the athlete's actions were unprofessional at best.

This incident of international importance (at least to the Paralympic Movement) certainly brought the issue of head injuries to the attention of many athletes. An important question needed to be asked about whether there is an advantage in competing against congenitally acquired cerebral palsy athletes for those who are head-injured through traumatic life experience. If individuals develop fine motor skills as a 'normal' person, they will acquire the muscle development that facilitates a well-functioning body. When people have the misfortune of suffering a head injury, certain muscles in the body may not function as they had done previously. No doubt loss of coordination may be an initial result, the degree of which is dependent upon the severity of the head injury. However, unlike the congenital cerebral palsy athlete, whose muscles never performed as they should (under 'normal' situations), the head-injured athlete will have some stored 'muscle memory' that it is believed advantages the athlete in terms of ability to perform. Therefore, the playing field is not level in terms of the classification of these two types of cerebral palsy athletes. The CP-ISRA might be able to rectify the anomaly by making an amendment to the classification system so that each of the eight classes has two distinct sub-classes, c for congenital and t for acquired through trauma. What is clear is that there needs to be sport science research to assess the validity of this proposition, because ethnographic evidence suggests c athletes are losing out to t athletes on a regular basis in sports such as cycling, where muscle memory can be seen as vital.

As to the reasons why the athlete was not expelled from the team, these remain unclear. One possible interpretation is that he was not given a life ban because he was a certainty when it came to winning gold medals.

In my view this case illustrates how serious the Paralympic Games had become. Medals were more important than anything else. Shortly after these Games the IPC took control over organising of the Games and the single sport world championships, and one of the first changes it implemented in the sport of athletics was that nations would be given places at the next Games based on the number of medals won at the last event. This meant that the number of medals won by each NPC became even more important. This is distinct to the way in which places are allocated in the Olympics, where a simple standard is the basis for selection in sports like athletics, with each country able to select three athletes for each event (and one relay team).[3] As a result of the IPC's decision, past performances by athletes who may no longer be on the team can determine whether there are enough places on a team for athletes who have met qualifying standards.

Such incidents did shift the culture within the Canadian Paralympic Committee, where they placed a great deal of emphasis on the team agreement that had to be signed before athletes, coaches and support staff were allowed to travel to an IPC-sanctioned event. At the same time other NPCs were requiring their athletes to sign similar documents in an attempt to manage the behaviour of their teams. Such controls may be seen as a product of the new professionalism in the sport that is believed to be closely linked with commercial pressures that are aimed at shaping it into a more marketable product. Codes of conduct are but one way in which the network of NPCs helps to guarantee the quality of the product in which the commercial organisations are investing.

Berlin 1994

By the time of the first IPCAC World Championships in Berlin during the summer of 1994, issues related to the power and influence of the IPC were on the minds of many of my like-minded fellow athletes. There were perhaps more people that I met and observed at this event than previously who were more concerned with securing improved sponsorship deals for themselves and therefore saw the 'professionalism' in the marketing of the IPC as being beneficial to their careers. The championships in Berlin were well organised, but they lacked the atmosphere and crowd support of the Paralympic Games. Perhaps athletics for the 'imperfect' was not something that captured the imagination of the German people, or the marketing of the IPC had not drawn the public's attention to the event. What is clear, from being present at the all IPCAC World Championships since then (1998, Birmingham, UK; 2002, Lille, France; and 2006, Assen, the Netherlands) is that none of these events seemed to draw much public support. Therefore, the limited interest in Berlin in 1994 is unlikely to be culturally specific.

Berlin in the summer of 1994 was the first time I publicly expressed my concern for the direction of the Paralympic Movement – first at an athletes' meeting and, in a more limited way, to various team officials and some of the members of the CP-ISRA that I had known since my first international involvement with sport for the disabled. One of many concerns both for members of the Canadian team as well as the British team (BBC 1994) was not the professional manner regarding how the championships were run, but rather who was allowed to compete in them. Athletes with learning impairments competed in an IPC-sanctioned event for the first time in Berlin, and there was real concern amongst the other athletes.

Many athletes with a disability have been stigmatised by their impairment. Such stigma can be a difficult burden and has a negative impact upon psychological and social well-being. Behind the stigma there is often the inherent feeling that 'if people get to know the real me' life will be better. Of course, things are not quite that simple. Everyone with an impairment is not a nice person, so the simple act of getting to know people is not always the answer. However, the issue that bothered many of the physically and sensory impaired athletes that had until now been the constituent members of the practice communitas (Howe and Jones 2006; see also Morgan 1994a) was that at home they had struggled to distance themselves from the tag 'Special Olympian'. The Special Olympics is an organisation which was established to give severely developmentally delayed individuals the opportunity to compete in sport. Traditionally each athlete gets a hug and a medal after competing, though there has been a shift in recent years toward an achievement model of sporting practice (Bale 1994). This was not the sporting ethos to which the new breed of Paralympian aspired. The athletes from the INAS-FID are not as impaired as those athletes who participate in the Special Olympics, as they do compete to win and, importantly, have some understanding of what that means.

This is the crux of the issue regarding INAS-FID athletes, and specifically those who participate in the Special Olympics. Why do they compete? Do they gain pleasure from training? These questions are relatively easy to answer for INAS-FID athletes, as my observations and interactions suggest that many of these athletes have been impaired in part by lack of integration and socialisation opportunities early in their development, and they appear keen and enthusiastic about their sport. On the other hand, Special Olympians appear to have very limited understanding of their sport or training, and it might be that the organisation was perhaps established as much for the parents and support staff involved with these individuals as for the athletes themselves. Their involvement can be seen as charitable, but because of the cognitive developmental level of many of the participants they could be simply going for a walk in the park on a sunny day rather than doing sport. It is this understanding of the Special Olympics and the image that it portrays regarding Paralympians that has given them cause for concern about the inclusion of the INAS-FID into the Paralympic Movement. Simply put, there is less perceived stigma associated with physical or sensory impairment than there is with an intellectual impairment. Therefore, the inclusion of the intellectually impaired was seen as an issue of grave concern to many of the athletes and IOSD officials during the summer of 1994. My observations from 1994 suggest that Paralympians ultimately are against the inclusion of the INAS-FID because Paralympic sport to them is concerned with the physical body, not with the mind. People with intellectual disabilities can perform at the level of mainstream professional sport and as a result they should seek these avenues for their competitive opportunities.[4]

Atlanta 1996

After the unprecedentedly successful Games in Barcelona in 1992, from the athletes' perspective the Games in Atlanta were a great disappointment. While competition was good, in the state-of-the-art Olympic venues the organisation was poor. The village that had been in place for the Olympic Games had been shut down. There was little in the way of entertainment – which to some might seem rather unproblematic, but with so much spare time on their hands during the Games before and between events athletes need distractions to help them unwind. Appropriate facilities were available for the Olympians, but the Para-lympians and 'their' organisations that lacked large corporate sponsorship were clearly not considered worthy of similar services. On one level we should cele-brate the lack of corporate involvement with the IPC because it suggests an organisation that does not desire to replicate the IOC, but at this juncture the reality is really quite different. Provision for entertainment had not been bud-geted at the Paralympic village by the local organising committee because they saw the running of the Paralympic Games as an annoyance. Not only was the village relatively cramped in terms of social space; the provision of cleaning ser-vices was also completely inadequate. As anyone who has lived in a Games village (Olympic or Paralympic) will attest, with so many people living on top of one another the rooms, washrooms and public spaces need to be cleaned very regularly. The village seemed to be cleaned once a week, and the dirt in the facilities is something that everyone who was in Atlanta village will no doubt remember less than fondly.

While the running of the competitions at the Atlanta Games appeared to be successful, transportation between the village and the stadium was extremely difficult. The organisers had brought in US marines to drive the accessible buses, and on several occasions after the system had been up and running for over a week I spent over an hour getting to the stadium on what should have been a fifteen-minute journey. Twice the driver had got lost, and on one occa-sion there were several competitors who missed the second call for their events and were lucky not to miss their event altogether. From the outside, there were some signs of optimism within the IPC. Atlanta marked the first time that the IPC had secured a global sponsor. The Coca-Cola® Corporation, with its inter-national headquarters in Atlanta, became a partner in the build-up to the 1996 Games. Such support from a major sponsor was a sign to the IPC that its organi-sation and the policies that established it were in fact working. It was in the same year that the first President of the IPC, in his full-time role of academic at the University of Alberta, writing to an academic audience, stated that there was a need to streamline classification used in the Paralympic Movement in order to help establish closer links with the IOC (Steadward 1996). Steadward's public discourse in his role as President of the IPC was less radical, but it can only be assumed that within the IPC executive these more radical views were part of free discussion as the Movement progressed toward his third and final term as President that began in 1997.[5] The fact that the Atlanta Games did not move the Paralympic Movement forward from the successes of Barcelona may have strengthened the resolve of the IPC to increase pressure on the sporting organisations such as the IPCAC to at least begin discussions on how classification could be streamlined within the sports.

The difficulties with the organisation of the Games and the impact that these had upon athletes in their preparations to perform, as well as a growing feeling that the IPC was travelling in a direction that would ultimately lead to the disempowering of certain classes of high-performance athletes with a disability, led me to pursue again a position as athletes representative on IPCAC. This role required me to represent the concerns of the athletes in the sport of track and field athletics. A relatively simple task, perhaps, but the position afforded no power to make decisions that would improve the lot for the most marginalised athletes within the IPC – those that were more severely impaired.

The decline in the number of Class 32 athletes who competed on the track was a personal concern. These athletes competed on the track by pushing their wheelchair with their feet (CP-ISRA 2001). In the mid-1980s there were track events at major Games for athletes in this class from 100 m to 800 m. At the Seoul Paralympics in 1988 there was a full complement of races on the programme for this classification, but four years later the interest of these athletes in track racing had seemingly disappeared. Class 32 athletes, whose upper body is less affected by athetosis, had continued to take an active part in field events. There was a concern within IPCAC that there were not enough of these athletes to run track events for them. The decline in numbers 'interested' in track racing also coincided with the development of the sport of Boccia as an event for a wide range of athletes with cerebral palsy, but particularly those were in CP-ISRA Classes 1 and 2.

Boccia is a game of skill that is scored in similar in the way to lawn bowling and in tournaments as well as World Championships and the Paralympic Games the events are run in a gymnasium. This game of skill, where players get points by being closer to the jack than their opponent, lacks the overt physicality of the track and field athletics, and as such does not in anyway make a spectacle of the bodies of the players. Boccia is a great game in its own right, requiring skill and tactical understanding, yet its lack of physicality means that the impaired bodies that play it do not get the health benefits of the training required to compete in track and field athletics. While this in itself is not a problem, because we should all be free to determine whether we should exercise, if lower cerebral-palsy classes were strong-armed out of the sport of track racing by political manoeuvring within the IPC then there are some important questions that need to be asked.

Another development that has occurred since 1994 has been an attempt to get these same athletes competing again on the track with a new mobility apparatus called a race runner. This is a support frame that has three wheels, like a tricycle without the chain, which athletes use to support their weight as they run around the track. The race runner was demonstrated at the 1994 and 1998 IPCAC World Championships as well as the Barcelona Paralympic Games, but has yet to be officially sanctioned as an official discipline within track athletics by the IPC. The reasons given are that it is still in the developmental stages as a discipline, and there seem to be few athletes interested in using a race runner to compete. Such criticism does have some validity. Certainly when the race runner was first developed in Denmark there were few athletes using it, and it was felt to be rather expensive to produce. Costs have since come down, and the issue of limited numbers of athletes is a self-fulfilling prophecy. The race runner was always demonstrated at athletic events where the athletes who would benefit from its inclusion as a viable discipline within the sport of track athletics were not present. Class 32 athletes who traditionally pushed their wheelchairs were no longer at the athletics venues during major events, as their class had been eliminated from the competition programme.

A politically astute move on the part of IPCAC would be to encourage a promotional team to carry our demonstrations of race runners during competitions run by the International Boccia Committee, whose athletes would benefit at least by its use as a recreational device. With increased exposure to the appropriate market we might soon see that some boccia players might enjoy the physicality of the race runner and, as a result, be eager to race it competitively. The step from here to having high- performance athletes training using the race runner is a much smaller one than that the IPCAC is requiring for those involved with the initiative to get the discipline included in the athletics programme at major events. Such efforts on the part of IPCAC would then send a clear message to the IPC that there are sports for the more severely impaired within their practice community (Morgan 1994a; Jones and Howe 2005), which may mean that the IPC does not need to invest efforts in establishing a specialised commission[6] for this group.

A seat at the IPCAC table

Through my role as athlete's representative I became acutely aware that most of the officials on the IPCAC were in these roles because they enjoyed organising international track and field meetings. The Chairman of the IPCAC was particularly good at this task, but seemed to lack the skills to delegate effectively. Part of the reason for this, of course, could be that all of the positions were filled by volunteers. The committee was made up of the Chair, Vice chair, Secretary, Treasurer, and Medical Officer, all of whom were elected by the nations at the IPCAC general assembly. The IOSDs each also had a member on the committee when I joined, but these were appointments made by the federations and the IPC was not particularly pleased that voting members of the

IPCAC were not elected by the nations.[7] It was the IOSD-appointed members who, at the first few meetings I attended, appeared to be have the most concern for the welfare of the athletes. A note related to a meeting held in February 1997 states:

> The tension in this meeting is quite extraordinary. I thought the committee members were all working to the same ends – providing good and equitable elite track meets. This does not seem to be the case and the group is really divided in three. First of all there is the group that is led by the chair that wishes to organise the most efficient meet and as a result issues related to equity appear to just annoy the group. The other group, led by the IBSA representative on the committee, is concerned with providing a good competition for his athletes. This faction also expressed concern that any competition needs to be equitable. Finally there were those individuals who appear to be here on a jolly at the expense of the IPC and seem to show little concern for any of the issues on the agenda other than issues related to expense claims.

These were the factions within the IPCAC that existed for the first two years of my tenure as athletes' representative. Committee members seemed to be reasonable people, but held very different understandings of the role of the committee.

Shortly after this meeting I aligned myself with the IBSA representative. The vision of this group (I use this term loosely, because at times it seemed to be two of us against the rest of the committee) was that athletics for the disabled should be well organised, but not to the point where athletes lose the opportunity to compete on a level playing field. As such, moves by the committee to implement changes to the classification system that were the result of long-term developments of the IOSDs seemed at best misguided. Simply put, those members of IOSDs that were concerned about issues related to equity felt that the classification systems were not negotiable. There were too few members of the committee who shared our vision, and as such the power base in the committee lay with the Chair and those individuals who wanted to organise athletics with little concern for the welfare of the athletes.

1998 IPC World Athletics Championships, Birmingham, UK

During the IPC Athletics World Championships, where I was present as a member of the committee (having been injured earlier in the season I was not fit enough to compete), I became increasingly concerned with the direction of the IPC and felt that I needed to attempt to move myself into a position where I could have more influence. Over the past two years it had become abundantly clear to me that the position of athletes' representative gave me a voice on the committee (and of course access to a fruitful research environment), but by and large it was a voice to which few on the committee paid any attention. Opinions from athletes for all IOSDs were gathered largely through email correspondence and information was disseminated to the committee. The desire of the committee to create the Steadward vision of high-performance sport for the disabled (Steadward 1996) that has close ties to the IOC began to overtake issues of equity within the practice communitas (Howe and Jones 2006).

During the Birmingham World Championships, an opportunity opened up as athletics technical officer for the CP-ISRA, the IOSD of which I was an athlete, and I decided to put my hat into the ring. There was an American international technical officer (a track and field official at the world championships) who was also interested in the post. The cultural capital that I had successfully cultivated over twelve years as a successful athlete and as an outspoken advocate facilitated my success in gaining the federation's nomination to the IPCAC. The sports technical committee of the CP-ISRA, of which I became a member, was a committee whose Chair had a seat on the executive committee of the federation. Each sport in which CP-ISRA athletes competed had a technical officer whose responsibility it was to liaise with organising committees about the sanctioning of federation events and to deal with questions and concerns, where appropriate, from the membership of the CP-ISRA. Of key importance was putting forward, and trying to win support for, the federation's view on issues relating to sports technical matters. It was my responsibility therefore to try, to the best of my ability, to put forward CP-ISRA views to the IPCAC and convince members that this was the best course of action. In practice, the negotiating that went on behind the scenes was never as clear-cut.

In hindsight, this minor victory of being made the CP-ISRA athletics technical officer at this stage backfired. As I had been elected to represent the athletes on the committee at the Atlanta 1996 Paralympic Games, and I could not wear two hats on the committee, the federation needed to deputise someone to represent the CP-ISRA until the next Paralympic Games in Sydney in 2000. The CP-ISRA appointed the American official, against whom I ran to get the post, to deputise for me. This was a mistake. The representatives of the IOSDs are charged with doing what is in the best interests of the constituent members, but this person appeared to have very limited understanding of the important issues in sport for the disabled and the CP-ISRA in particular. While he was supposed to take a lead from me on decisions, he was unsupportive and I believe this may have been a factor in the loss of votes that are still having an effect on the athletes in the CP-ISRA.

A case in point is the development of decathlon-style tables for the throwing events. These tables were established using the results of throwing events at the Birmingham World Championships. By taking the three medallists' distances and the current world record and adding them all together and then dividing by four, the distance obtained was considered to be worth 1000 points. Performances for an athlete in a given class could have their success measured against this mark. In the eyes of the committee this approach could facilitate competition not only between athletes within different classes in the same disability group but also across the IOSDs. The benefit of this system as far as the IPC was concerned (and those in the IPCAC who were concerned with organising well-oiled athletics matches) was that events could be staged combining numerous classes, and thus streamlining the programme. To the committee and the practice communitas, these tables were portrayed as a way of safeguarding events for athletes who would not otherwise have a viable competition at the major championships. With the implementation of the IPC rule that there must be six athletes from four different countries, there was fear from some quarters that there needed to be a solution to save events. In practice, however, the system has led to the further reduction of competitive opportunities for the athletes who need them most. By adopting the tables on a rolling two-year cycle, where results at the World Championships help create the tables used at the Paralympic Games and then the Paralympic results are used to create the tables for the World Championships, it means that, standards, which are also based on the tables, vary depending on how the medal winners performed at the last major championship. If a class of medallist performs brilliantly well, then the standard for the next World Championship or Paralympic Games will be very high, as 1000 points will be a greater distance and therefore the class may struggle to get enough athletes to qualify with the A standard so that they can eventually have an event that is viable in its own right, without the necessity to combine it with another class(es) and or disability group.

IPC Athletic Committee and performance tables

The IPCAC as a political body runs the sport of athletics through performance tables. By and large the IOSDs, the founding members of the IPC, consider this inappropriate. In the case of the IBSA, they opted not to use tables for the reason that it was not in the spirit of track and field athletics. As a result, when the blind athletes do not have enough athletes to run competitions they will combine classes within the federation, using the same standards for all athletes in a combined class, and the event is run in the same way as the less-impaired event. If, however, there are enough of the more impaired class to have an event on their own, then the less-impaired athletes will be excluded from the event.

Tensions were at a high point within the IPCAC in the lead-up to the Sydney 2000 Games with regard to the debate surrounding the use of tables. For a time it made meetings of the committee less than productive, with the three factions opposed to one another. The lack of agreement that surrounded the issue of decathlon tables was part of the broader debate surrounding classification. Since the tables effectively eliminated events from the programme, they were seen positively by the IPCAC Chair. The argument ran that the tables actually saved events, but in reality they changed the nature of the competition. By rating performances on a scale (the decathlon tables), athletes involved in field events could theoretically compete against any athlete from any IOSD. As a reason for establishing equitable competition, degree of impairment was considered to be of little importance. With the exception of the athletes from the IBSA, whose federation opted out of the use of tables, all potential Paralympians could compete in the same field event. Running one shot-put competition for men instead of over fifteen[8] reduces the logistical challenges of scheduling multiple shot competitions.

In reality, the IPCAC has not as yet streamlined the programme in this way. Field events are being staged as if there are enough athletes to meet the general IPC rule that there must be six athletes from four nations. In 2000, the committee added the caveat that for an event to be viable there must be ten athletes of a 'good' standard on each class's IPC ranking list. While the IPCAC equates a 'good' standard with a close competition where athletes are producing results of a similar standard, such a stance does not consider the specific nature of impairment. The IAAF does not make similar decisions in terms of the events that it runs at major championships. The great Ukrainian pole vaulter Sergey Bubka was, in the late 1980s and early 1990s, setting world records that were twenty centimetres higher than his fellow competitors could manage, yet the IAAF would never consider cancelling the pole vault because it was uncompetitive. Because the IPCAC does not define what is meant by a competitive competition it is in the powerful position of being able to determine which events are run at major championships. Unless a class can get the IPC regulated number of athletes over the IPCAC A standard, the committee is entitled to combine the class with another. The act of combining classes artificially increases the standards for each class in the combined event because NPCs are less likely to see athletes in combined events unless tables work to their advantage.

Difficulties also arise when classes are combined across IOSDs because the IPCAC assumes they are equivalent and therefore the use of tables is seen as inappropriate. In recent years this has happened with Classes F51 and F32. In Class 51, the 5 signifies that the athlete is classified by IWAS and therefore is a wheelchair user. This class means that the athlete has suffered a cervical lesion with complete or incomplete quadriplegia (DePauw and Gavron 1995), and the result of this type of impairment is that the athlete lacks the ability to generate much power through their body. Athletes that comprise Class 32 are classified by the CP-ISRA. These Class 2 athletes are also quadriplegic accompanied by poor functional strength in all extremities and trunk, but have the ability to propel a wheelchair. Class 32 athletes have a degree of strength that is greater than the Class 51 athletes, but lack the ability to control this due to severe spasticity. 'Upper extremity athletes with athetosis may demonstrate fair rotation during throwing with unreliable release. In athletes with spasticity or athetosis the trunk makes a very limited contribution to propulsion of the implement' (CP-ISRA 2001: 30). From the outside it may appear that because both classes of athletes are quadriplegic, their impairment must be very similar. The literal meaning of quadriplegia is the state of having paralysis in all four limbs, but the nature of the paralysis is distinct and it is a lack of understanding of the individual impairment that has resulted in the IPCAC placing these classes together without the use of tables.

The issue of appropriate use of taxonomy in the classification process is brought to the fore by Tweedy (2002) in his attempt to begin the debate regarding a unified disability athletics classification. Tweedy (2002: 229) has argued that by using the language of the International Classification of Functioning, Disability and Health (ICF) we would be able to move away from some of the ambiguities that exist when comparing the classification systems of the CP-ISRA, ISMWSF and ISOD:

> The clarity and effectiveness of the eligibility criteria are compromised by the use of terms that are not standardised, such as 'functionally be equated' (ISMWSF system), 'similar conditions' (CP-ISRA system), and 'resembling' (ISOD amputee system).
>
> (Tweedy 2002: 229)

There is a degree of difficulty in determining what each IOSD actually means by each of these phrases. In their attempts to combine classes the IPCAC may have been taking the ambiguous statements at face value, but, as Tweedy warns, 'it is surely a matter of debate as to which disabilities can functionally be equated with spinal cord injury' (2002: 229). In the meetings that I attended there was considerable heated debate over the means by which events should be combined, but few of the committee saw such discourse as politically charged. To most of the IPCAC those of us who were 'being difficult', in our opposition to integrated classification systems, were seen as not being aware of how to run a good track and field athletics meeting.

The minefield that needed to be crossed at every meeting was made more difficult by the structuring of meetings so that opportunities for debate on issues related to the best interest of the athletes were marginalised. Agendas were established to limit the 'trouble makers' from derailing the meetings. On numerous occasions during my seven-year tenure on the committee I was taken aside and lobbied by the Chair about one thing or another in an attempt to win my support for an important vote. Early on as an athletes' representative I began to realise that the responsibility of the job was to stand up for the more marginalised athletes within the remit of the IPCAC, yet this stance made me relatively unpopular. My main concern was that athletes should have an opportunity to compete on the world stage regardless of their level of impairment, and the fact that I was less concerned with the numbers in severely impaired classes meant that my tenure as the athletes representative was not an easy one. The IPCAC for its part as happy for events to go ahead for the severely impaired and for women (who can be seen in the context of sport for the disabled to be marginalised; see Chapter 8) if there was an appropriate number of competitors. However, in many cases events for these athletes did not have enough competitors and thus were removed from the Paralympic or World Championship programme. Once eliminated from the programme of a major event the chances of the event being run again are very slim, as events run at the previous championship (either the Paralympics or the IPC Worlds) are the cornerstone for the next programme. As a result, the programme gets smaller and smaller.

There is an assumption within the IPCAC that if there are only a couple of athletes in a class then they are not elite. Ironically, a greater number of competitors in a race or field event cannot be used as a determinant of elite status. Big city marathons such as London or New York have over 25 000 competitors each year, but as few as thirty of these would be considered elite athletes if performance were the key consideration. No doubt some classes may adopt a more elite approach to training and competition as a result of wanting to be better than others in their class; however, numbers and similar quality of performance should not be the only factor used to determine whether a particular event has an elite status.

Being an elite athlete is not simply synonymous with involvement in high-performance sport. High performance suggests that a competitor is very close to what has been pre-determined by past achievements in a sporting practice as being at the physical limits of the event, and this may be distinct from elite status. Elite status can be defined as the intensive and long-term commitment to training and competition. Therefore, an athlete who lacks certain physical skills could be seen to be an elite performer simply by embodying the habitus of other elite performers. This entails making sacrifices both socially and physically that are part of the cultural capital that elite athletes hold. In the majority of the sporting world high-performance athletes and elite athletes are one and the same; however, in relatively new sporting practices such as women's pole vault and steeplechase, where a limited number of athletes have been drawn to the events only relatively recently, it is hard to determine where the status of high performance begins. With world records being set in the women's pole vault almost at will during the time of writing by one athlete who is head and shoulders better than the rest (Yelena Isinbayeva of Russia), this event is not that dissimilar to events run with very few competitors at the Paralympics or the IPC Athletics World Championships. The IPCAC has attempted to avoid the criticism of the cancellation of field events by adopting the use of tables highlighted earlier, but in reality once events are combined the chance of them being split again are not great. Ultimately, the use of the decathlon tables has facilitated the streamlining of the athletics programme while externally suggesting the IPCAC is working to preserve competitive opportunities for more severely impaired and female athletes, who are more likely to be involved in events that are forced to adopt the use of tables.

The simplest measure of whether a disability classification is interested in a particular sporting opportunity is to look at the ranking lists that are now annually (if not more regularly) updated by members of the technical committee. The IPCAC continually makes decisions about events to include in its competitive programme based on two specific statistics – the number of athletes on the ranking lists and how close or competitive their performances are as a classification. For sports technical committees such as the IPCAC, the decision to eliminate events is relatively easy. While constituent members representing the IOSDs continually express concern over their athletes losing out on high-profile competitive opportunities, the decision to eliminate events is celebrated behind closed doors as it facilitates the move to a more simplistic programme which is easier to organise. It is not surprising that sport technical committees such the IPCAC work toward this goal. Since the Barcelona Paralympics of 1992, the sport of swimming has been held up as a model of good practice by some (Daly and Vanlandewijck 1999; Drummer 1999) for providing a simple clear classification system, and as a flawed system by others (Richter *et al.* 1992; Martin *et al.* 1995; Wu *et al.* 2000), since ultimately the act of streamlining the swimming classification system appears to have been done in the best interest of the sport and not in the best interest of the athletes.

What is most worrying is that most of the members of the IPCAC are not aware of the political importance of the decisions they are making on behalf of the athletes. It also seems that the NPCs agree that IPCAC moves to stream-line the sport of athletics are in the best interest of the athletes. At the 2002 general assembly, NPCs passed a motion that removes the IOSDs from the IPCAC and replaces them with members at large elected by the NPCs. In many respects this might mean the end of the politically motivated discussions born out of advocacy, which may in time lead to a more productive committee – but to what end? Who will speak for the athletes, since the role of their representa-tive will be increasingly marginalised in light of the new committee structure? Most of the IOSD members with whom I have worked on this committee, either as athletes' representative or an IOSD member myself, loosely believed in providing good competitive opportunities for their athletes and seldom seemed concerned how smoothly the programme of events ran at the Paralympics or World Championships.

IPC Athletics Committee culture

It was suggested in the previous section that IPCAC was roughly divided into three political factions. Those individuals who were largely concerned with organising an elite track and field athletics meeting were by and large the power behind the committee, as they were elected at the general assembly of the NPCs. The second group, consisting of a number of appointed representatives from the IOSDs and the athletes' representative, were primarily concerned with facilitating opportunities for their athletes to perform in world-class events. Other members of the group were often present because they enjoyed the inter-national free travel, and seldom seemed to be either prepared for the meetings, except when it came to claiming expenses. This dynamic at the committee meetings meant that members that were just pleased to be away from grind of daily life actually held often-pivotal positions and deciding votes.

The social environment that this committee's culture created was at times not conducive to moving forward the sport of athletics, partly because the various factions of the committee seemed to disagree on the future of IPC ath-letics. The power base was largely held by the Chair, who was initially involved in the sport through the ISMWSF (and later the IWAS) but, because this was a stronger federation, largely based upon the number of athletes in any one class, issues regarding whether events needed to be saved seldom registered on his radar. Some of the appointed members from the IOSDs felt that the goal of running a smooth, well-oiled track and field meet was not the only aim of the committee. Higher goals are also the aim of the Paralympic Movement.

Currently, for example, the motto of the IPC is 'Spirit in Motion'. According to the IPC, 'The word "Spirit" is derived from the notion that the IPC, like the athletes it represents, has a drive to compete and to succeed' (IPC 2003a: 1). Motion, on the other hand, 'relates to the fact that the IPC is truly moving forward – an organisation that realises its potential and is now striving to achieve it' (IPC 2003a: 1). While changes have taken place within the IPCAC, whether they are truly progressive steps is unclear. What is certain is that athletes are not any closer to being in a positions of influence within the IPCAC then they were over a decade ago.

The development of the new logo and motto for the IPC marks a new chapter in the Movement of which the IPCAC with no ties to the IOSD cultural baggage will be a part. As with any organisation's logo, the elaboration by the organisation itself never clarifies the intent. In fact, the shift from the old to the new logo (see Figure 3.1) explicitly suggests that physical movement of the athlete is of particular importance. According to the IPC website,[9]

> The new Paralympic Symbol consists of three elements in red, blue and green – the three colours that are most widely represented in national flags around the world. It is a symbol that is in motion, with three Agitos (from the Latin word 'agito', meaning 'I move') encircling a centre point; emphasizing the role that the IPC has of bringing athletes from all corners of the world together and enabling them to compete.

This of course facilitates equity between able and disabled athletes regardless of impairment, since traditionally physicality is fundamental to the sporting enterprise (DePauw 1997), and as such sporting participants with an impairment have traditionally been overshadowed as a result of a lack of ability in comparison with their 'able' peers.

Observations taken over the past two decades suggest that the shift in motto is nothing more that a marketing exercise. In fact, the Spirit in Motion motto sits uneasily with the vision of the IPC launched at the same time on 5 April 2003. The vision of the IPC is 'To Enable Paralympic Athletes to Achieve Sporting Excellence and to Inspire and Excite the World' (IPC 2003a: 1). Clearly this has an embodied element associated with it that the new motto does not. Working alongside a marketing team, the IPC Executive Committee, along with many IPC stakeholders, developed this new image (IPC 2003a: 1). It is ironic therefore that, with all this forward thinking and movement, the same issue of *The Paralympian* discusses the establishment of the IPC Commission for Athletes with a Severe Disability (CASD), which was formed in October 2002

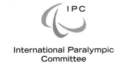

Figure 3.1 Paralympic logo 2003–present. © International Paralympic Committee.

(IPC 2003a: 6). If the IPC were doing all it could for its constituent members, surely the most important of which are the severely impaired athletes, since they often struggle to find appropriate sporting opportunities in the mainstream, then the forward-thinking organisation that the IPC professes to be would not need to have a special commission to represent the concerns of any of its athletes. An athlete with a severe disability[10] is either a person who requires assistance during competition that is allowed through the rules of a sport, or a person who requires a carer for daily living functions.

The struggle within the IPC between groups with apparently similar objectives is partly what makes the culture of the IPCAC distinctive. Elected members of the committee, most of whom are dedicated to running an efficient track and field meeting, appointed members of the various IOSDs in large part looking to enhance the quality of their constituent members sporting experience, and various hangers on tend to battle in the political forum. Battles for control of the sport of athletics were waged in person at quarterly meetings, but by and large the positioning of the battle lines was established in one of two ways: through communications (usually electronically) from the Chair to committee members, and also by an absence of the same. When the Chair felt that a decision was likely to be controversial, he might wait until the last possible minute to inform committee members that a decision needed to be reached in a few days. To control the IPCAC, decisions of significance were often taken by only a few members of the committee – the reason given being that members (often the those representing the IOSDs) had to respond to the call for information. Often the members of the committee representing IOSDs were unable to solicit opinions from their members at such short notice because all officials within the CP-ISRA were unpaid volunteers who have other roles and responsibilities and, as a result, cannot turn their hand to federation business at very short notice. In the autumn of 2001, notes reflecting on a communication I had with the Chair reflect some of my frustration:

> It has happened again. A plea from IPCAC for information – yesterday. Why could such a request not be dealt with at the next meeting? The Chair says that timeline has been set by the IPC so that it was not up to him. There is almost two years until the Games in Sydney and he is already asking for clarification of viable events from the federation. Some athletes of a high calibre now could have reached elite status in a year's time and be ready to challenge for honours in Oz. How can I stop the steamroller? Why is there no time following a IPC World Athletics Championships for the IOSDs to take stock of the situation? It seems that IPCAC wants only viable events at the last IPC event to be included in the next. This is strong-arming us (CP-ISRA) into limiting the opportunity for our athletes and really places a dampener on any development programmes.

Such events were not uncommon during my seven-year tenure on the committee. Confrontation between the various factions of the group was inevitable as a direct result of the management style and motivation of the Chair. What lay behind much of the orchestrating of the arguments of the committee may have been a latent paternalism on part of some of the constituent members of the IPC more generally.

This paternalism by and large is rooted in the notion that a lack of physicality requires rehabilitation towards a normative goal. It was of course the principle of rehabilitation that led Sir Ludwig Guttmann to organise the first Games for spinal cord-injured individuals following the Second World War (DePauw and Gavron 1995; Seymour 1998), yet the Western emphasis of the physically normal individual is someone who needs to be helped. Certainly the role of medical understanding of impairments has gone a long way in shaping the political culture surrounding disability (Oliver 1990), and this can be seen to have impacted upon sport in the disabled communitas. Issues of disability have been considered problematic in the West (Edgerton 1976; Whyte and Ingstad 1995). Sporting practices that were originally established to facilitate rehabilitation to a normative existence were seen as a method of dealing with the social problems associated with impairment. As a result, paternalistic attitudes are prevalent within the sport for the disabled communitas.

Since sport is a Western construct, it is perhaps not surprising that its provision for the disabled communitas is also has its foundation in the West. As such the relationship between politics and disability has an impact on how sport for the disabled has developed, and it is to this that the next chapter now turns.

4 The politics of sporting disablement

The previous chapter highlights some of the lived experiences I have had within the Paralympic Movement, many of which have been overtly political, such as my membership on various committees. This chapter will explore the political explicitly in sport for the disabled. In order to achieve this aim the chapter will begin by examining the politics of disability, and draws on key thinkers in order to establish the relationship between people with impairments and how they are understood within the mainstream. From here we will turn to the Foucauldian concept of governmentality as it has been used within the field of sports studies. The adoption of governmentality is salient here, since it allows an understanding of the politics of controlling the body and therefore is appropriate when considering the process of disablement (Verbrugge and Jette 1994). The chapter finishes with a detailed discussion of classification in sport for the disabled, since this process is overtly political.

The politics of disability

In his landmark work *The Politics of Disablement* (1990), Oliver makes a conscious attempt at formulating a social understanding of disablement based on the theoretical insights of Marx and Weber. Though sport for the disabled does not feature in the text, the argument highlights that the Western construction of disability is an individual medicalistic problem, which enables society at large to firmly control the members of the disabled communitas. This work made a vital contribution to allowing social scientists to re-evaluate the research on disability from a critical though increasingly unfashionable perspective. With the advent of post-modern and post-structural accounts of identity formation (Riddell and Watson 2003a), traditional structural analysis has fallen out of favour. However, a collective understanding of a communitas still has value in attempting to determine if there are common experiences that are shared.

> The hegemony that defines disability in a capitalist society is constituted by the organic ideology of individualism, the arbitrary ideologies of medicalisation underpinning medical intervention and personal tragedy theory

underpinning much social policy. Incorporated also are ideologies related to the concepts of normality, able-bodiedness and able-mindedness.

(Oliver 1990: 44)

Therefore, if research were to abandon an agenda for equality and the redistribution of goods and services in favour of a focus upon diversity and difference, we might find ourselves in a situation where there is a lack of critique of the structural inequalities that may impact upon how the disabled communitas can be represented (Riddell and Watson 2003b: 2). I am not suggesting here that individual identity is not important, as the second half of this monograph will attest; rather, individual identity, which in the case of Paralympic athletes is partly determined by type and degree of impairment, is less significant when looking at organisations such as the IPC.

Oliver (1990) ties the transformation of the economy during the industrial revolution to the institutionalisation of the disabled. With the shift from a rural to an urban environment there was a need to 'remove' the physically disabled from their homes, since they were not seen as having the ability actively to contribute to the economic viability of the family home. The physical removal of the disabled from their homes and their emergence in large numbers in institutional setting meant that they became marginalised as a result. This adoption of a historical materialist account focusing upon the medical classification of disabilities according to functional categories would lead to a better curative environment if each institution specialised in rehabilitating specific groups.

For scholars within the multidisciplinary field of disability studies, Oliver's analysis led to the conceptualisation of disability as a social constraint. The resulting 'social model of disability', developed from the 1960s but brought to a wider audience in the publication *Fundamental Principles of Disability* (UPIAS 1976), was a political statement of intent by the Union of the Physically Impaired Against Segregation. Highlighted through the work of Oliver (1990), this approach sees disability as an individual medicalistic problem which, as stated above, enables society at large to firmly control the members of the impaired communitas (Oliver and Barnes 1998; Thomas 1999):

> In our view, it is society which disables physically impaired people. Disability is something imposed on top of our impairments by the way we are unnecessarily isolated and excluded from participation in society. Disabled people are therefore an oppressed group.
>
> (Oliver 1996: 22)

If disability is a social construction, a product of medicalisation, as those who advocate a social model of disability suggest, it is perhaps not surprising that so little attention within disability studies has been paid to the practice of sport, which has traditionally classified bodies on medical grounds.

The category of disability

The notion of the categorisation of impairments that leads directly to a marginal position in society stems from the work of Erving Goffman (1963). Categorising the body based on its degree of difference places it on a continuum where one trait may make an individual less marginalised than someone else who exhibits another different trait. *Stigma: Some Notes on the Management of Spoiled Identity* (Goffman 1963) was one of the first studies that drew attention to the nature of the problem of the stigmatisation of people with impairments. Some critics (Oliver 1990; Barnes 1991) have argued that the role of studies of stigma was an attempt to medicalise disability in order to classify it in respect to the predominate views that are expressed by society at large. For this reason, Goffman's work on stigma is useful when exploring the categorisation (or rather classification) of athletes with a disability. After all, the practice of classifying for sport is largely a medical one that can lead to stigmatisation and alienation because it ultimately creates a hierarchy of bodies. Turner's conceptualisation of 'liminality' (1967, 1969) is also useful, since it positions stigmatised individuals at the margins of society. Murphy (1987) suggests

> 'Betwixt and Between' is actually a neat description of the ambiguous of the disabled.... The long-term physically impaired are neither sick nor well, neither dead nor fully alive, neither out of society nor wholly in it. They are human beings but their bodies are warped or malfunctioning, leaving their full humanity in doubt. They are not ill, for illness is transitional to either death or recovery. Indeed, illness is a fine example of nonreligious, nonceremonial liminal condition. The sick person lives in a state of social suspension until he or she gets better. The disabled spend a lifetime in a similar suspended state.
>
> (Murphy 1987: 131)

There are problems with seeing people with disabilities as being entirely marginalised, since this suggests that the social position of the disabled communitas hinges upon concepts such as 'symbolic order' (Douglas 1966). The concept of liminality illuminates the position of the disabled communitas, in society. In order to improve the position of the disabled communitas those working within disability studies have adopted an emancipatory paradigm. To avoid further oppression for the disabled communitas by the able-bodied mainstream, emancipatory research is an approach that Barnes suggests is important:

> Emancipatory research is about the systematic demystification of the structures and processes which create disability, and the establishment of a workable 'dialogue' between the research communit[as] and the disabled people in order to facilitate the latter's empowerment.
>
> (Barnes 1992: 122)

This approach to research is explicitly politically driven, and is implicitly at the heart of this monograph – as Charlton (1998) has suggested in the title of his thought-provoking work, *Nothing about Us Without Us*. In order to achieve this aim it is useful to explore the work of the social theorist, Michel Foucault, which offers further salience to a discussion regarding categorisation of various bodies (Foucault 1977).

Importantly, Foucault's work can be used to explore classification within sport for the disabled. The work of Foucault has been shown by scholars working in the field of sport studies to provide an appropriate critique of the objectification of the sporting body, particularly as it relates to scientific classification and dividing practices (Markula and Pringle 2006: 25–26). The process of classifying an athlete for involvement within the Paralympic Games, for example, may be seen as the scientific classification of an organism that ultimately leads in some way to its marginalisation – being separated from the social environment because of the distinctive nature of classification and the manner in which Paralympic sport is practised. This act of classification is overtly political, since processing of the body into a particular class is a form of segregation. In order to make sense of the political transformations within elite sport for the disabled, this chapter will outline Foucault's conceptualisation of governmentality.

Foucault's governmentality

'Governmentality' is term used to link the body of work regarding technologies of discipline found in *The Birth of the Clinic* (Foucault 1973) and *Discipline and Punish* (Foucault 1977), for example, and Foucault's later work on sexuality that more explicitly focuses upon the technologies of the self (Markula 2003; Smith-Maguire 2003). Governmentality is a useful way of exploring the control that social institutions have over individuals within society. Governmentality 'incorporates both techniques or practices of self-government and the more apparent forms of external government – policing, surveillance and regulatory activities carried out by agencies of the state or other institutions for strategic purposes' (Lupton 1995: 9). In other words, society uses individual consciousness to perpetuate the system. Individual choice is as important as the structure of society. More explicitly, governmentality for Foucault 'refers to a "mentality" or way of thinking about the administration of society, in which the population is managed through the beliefs, needs, desires, and choices of individuals' (Smith-Maguire 2003: 307).

The process of classification within sport for the disabled is perhaps the most important manner in which athletes are governed. The approaches taken by individual IOSDs vary, partly because some of the impairments are sensory and others are physical, but the principles behind the advent of each system are the same – the creation of an equitable sporting environment. Detailed discussion of the systems of classification within the sports of athletics and swimming has occurred elsewhere (Howe 2006b; Howe and Jones 2006), but the cultural political environment surrounding the process has not, and I believe the work of Foucault and that of scholars who have engaged with it (Andrews 1993; Rail and Harvey 1995; Smith-Maguire 2002; Markula 2003; Cole *et al.* 2004; Markula and Pringle 2006) can help to address this lacuna.

The work of Foucault is not only linked to the body but also the associated issues of power and the knowledge construction. Like most scholars, Foucault's project shifted focus throughout his lifetime. His early work was concerned with the technologies of dominance, and it is the work that has the most salience when exploring sport for the disabled. The subsequent sections will begin by exploring the technologies of dominance, before turning attention to the process of classification in an attempt to lay the foundation for the exploration of the politics of Paralympic sport from the position of Foucault's governmentality.

Technologies of dominance

In the wider social sciences, the conceptualisations of the individual body as a vessel ripe for manipulation, the social body (Turner 1992, 1996) and the body politic (Scheper-Hughes and Lock 1987; Lock 1993) can be seen to be influenced by Foucault. Because of the habitual nature of training within sporting environments, whether individuals train and compete as a member of a team or perform in sport which is individual in nature (such as track and field athletics or golf), the elite performer often has a support team (including medical staff, coaches, etc.) which provides a social environment distinctive to that sport (Shogun 1999). The social environment where training of sporting participants takes place, then, whether for a team or as an individual, is where the disciplined body can be seen to be developed. The conceptualisation of the socially disciplined body that Foucault (1977) articulates has also been, in one form or other, and perhaps unconsciously, a focus for good coaches' training procedures for generations (Park 1992).

The need for coaches to control the training regimes of their athletes so that the embodied athlete performs to the best of his or her ability is something that increased as sporting practice transformed from being considered a leisure pastime to being a professional concern where a winning result was linked to economic gain (Howe 2004a). Following a rigid training regime, the power to dominate the development of the sporting body can be seen as an extension of the genealogy[1] that is the foundation of the Foucaudian method. Archaeology is an elementary form of Foucault's method of genealogy (a moment of interpretation) which both examines historical antecedents as well as the analysis of the emergence of discourse. The genealogy is an interpretative strategy that is distinctive from traditional history. As Andrews (1993: 156) suggests, the development of disciplinary practice

> revolved around the emergence of a cluster of disciplinary institutions which, in terms of structure and ideology, promoted the ethos of discipline. Institutions such as prisons, hospitals, and schools increasingly came to the

fore, augmented by complementary structures of knowledge and related human sciences that rationalized and legitimated the agenda of social discipline.

Sport today, particularly the way in which coach–athlete relationships are structured, can clearly be seen as a disciplinary institution, where the athletes body is in part controlled through the training process (Pronger 2002).

The technologies of domination and principally the act of discipline are important in examining sporting contexts such as sporting practices for the disabled, because they develop a distinctive form of power that may be seen as tools which control the body not in an oppressive manner but rather with the aim of normalising it (Rail and Harvey 1995: 165). Following on from this point, Cole *et al.*(2004: 212) state:

> [B]odies are never simply trained but are subjected to normative judgments (which include an ethical dimension), or what Foucault called divided practices. At least dividing practices are forces of 'normalisation' that produce and exclude through reference to a norm. Techniques of normalisation distinguish the normal from the pathological, or the normal from the threatening.

This act of normalisation that is part of society generally has had an influence on research within the field of disability studies, particularly when related to service provision for people with a disability (Tyne 1992: 34), where normalisation can be seen as a good thing if it leads to the empowerment of members of the disables communitas. The adoption of 'care in the communitas' as a primary vehicle for the assimilation or normalisation of people with impairments can be seen have had an impact upon the way in which sporting practices for the disabled have developed. Research conducted by Williams (1994a, 1994b) suggests that sporting practice is a useful way to socialise individuals with disabilities. But socialisation to what end? The process of normalisation to people who physically lack normality can be problematic. In what way are they socialised? If socialisation just occurs in the limited world of sport for the disabled, has the goal of integration been achieved?

It is clear that able and disabled 'bodies are invested with power relations, making them the legitimate target of the interventions of medicine, education and economics' (Smith-Maguire 2002: 299). In other words, technologies of dominance shape the world in and around sport for the disabled, and perhaps are even more apparent at the high-performance end of the spectrum. While this maybe the case in some respects, the key technology of dominance in the world of disabled sport is the classification system, which at once illuminates the nexus between the means of disciplining the individual body and those of the population as a whole. Before turning to classification within sport for the disabled, we should first turn our attention toward the process of classification.

Process of classification

The culture that surrounds sporting practice and the knowledge participants have of their bodies and their self-identity means that to work towards achieving goals on an individual level is just as important as the work done through and by institutions:

> Through work on and with the body, we experience, establish, and extend our limits and abilities, while placing them in the context of a number of rules and styles that make up our social circumstances. This is not simply a matter of doing exercises, but of monitoring and refining, keeping training records and making confessions, giving and taking up different behaviours.
>
> (Smith-Maguire 2002: 303)

This in a sense is a form of self-surveillance that all elite athletes go through. In this regard, the world of the elite sport for the disabled is indistinguishable from the sporting mainstream except for the process of classification. While other sporting practices have forms of classification (such as by age and weight), because the general population varies across the categories they are less restrictive than the protocols established by the IOSDs where classification is impairment specific.

Whether the advent of a new system will improve on the old impairment-specific classification is unclear. Critics of the relatively new integrated classification system suggest that some impairment groups maybe at a systematic disadvantage, and in some cases no longer able to compete (McCann 1994; Richter 1994). Specifically, the system may be more difficult to classify because of the need to consider a great number of impairments simultaneously, and many of the tests used have not been statistically validated (Richter *et al.* 1992). There is a fear that some athletes will 'cheat' the system by fooling the classifiers because the classification tests have not been validated statistically. According to Wu and Williams (1999: 262):

> Misclassification is an interesting and perennial problem in disability sport. As with many others, it is the root cause of much frustration and anger (a) among swimmers who feel they have been disadvantaged by losing to a competitor who should be in a higher class and (b) among coaches and swimmers who may believe that they have been disadvantaged by being placed in a higher class than their impairment warrants.

Perhaps most importantly, athletes may be penalised for enhancing their own performance. Athletes who train and improve their technique in swimming (or any sport that adopts an integrated functional classification system) may be reclassified based on their new ability. This is a key concern:

> The concept of athletic excellence can only be fully appreciated when the performance is related to the functional physical resources available to the

athlete in competition. These resources represent the athlete's performance potential. Whether such a potential is fully utilized by the athlete is one crucial determinant of excellence. An acceptable classification system would allow the definition and measurement of performance potential. The definition of *potential* in this way is the cornerstone of the classification process.

(Vanlandewijck and Chappel 1996: 73)

In practice, the determination of sporting potential is almost impossible to achieve through any of the current classification systems in place in Paralympic sport. Yet the aim of achieving as fair a competition as possible is still the goal of the classification process.

On another level, the body of an athlete is also controlled by sports governing bodies which act as administrative and bureaucratic centres with ever-increasing commercial agendas (see Chapter 5). Currently the IPC is eager to win control of the classification process for all its sports, which will ultimately lead to the implementation of a Code of Practice by the end of 2007. The IPC suggests 'The classification code will aim to synchronise all sport specific classification processes and procedures, in much the same way that the world Anti-Doping Code has done for international anti-doping rules and regulations' (IPC 2004: 11).

Governmentality and the Paralympic Movement

Ludwig Guttmann, the father of the Paralympic Movement (see Chapter 2), was clear that it was classification that was the distinctive component of governance within sport for the disabled.

> rules must necessarily be combined with correct classification according to the extent of physical deficit to ensure fair play, and such classifications have been compiled over the years in co-operation with panels of medical and technical experts ... in the various fields of disablement.
>
> (Guttmann 1976, Preface)

The pace of transformation of sport for the disabled from its roots in rehabilitative medicine to high-performance sport has been dramatic. The social environment in which sport for the disabled exists has been transformed more rapidly than any sporting practice in history. Since 1989, when the IPC was established, there has been a constant push within the organisation to achieve a level footing with the International Olympic Committee (IOC) (Mason 2002; Howe and Jones 2006). The move from a foundation in rehabilitation (DePauw and Gavron 1995; Seymour 1998) into the realm of achievement sports (Bale 2004) can been seen to have shaped development of sport for the disabled not only at the level of the international sporting spectacle, but also right the way through to the grassroots. The governance by the IOSDs, with their mandate for elite as well as grassroots sport, want to see a 'level playing field'.

Classification is a good example of governmentality, since the nexus between technologies of the self and of dominance is fundamental because the relationships between the means of disciplining the individual body and regulating a population are key and important. Some scholars have suggested that '[c]lassification, sociologically, can be conceptualised as a mechanism for positive social control in that it provides both the structure and the process for operationalising' (Wu *et al*. 2000: 420) sport for the disabled. This functionalist understanding of classification belies the fact that social control can also have negative connotations. While research does suggest that classifiers do maintain one of the most important systems in disabled sport (Richter *et al*. 1992; Vanlandewijck and Chappel 1996; Sherill 1999), the assumption that control they exert is a good thing needs to be examined.

Politically, classification was and still is a contested terrain. Classification is a process that athlete's bodies must go through in order to be involved in Paralympic sport, and therefore is not dissimilar to the weighing of boxers before they fight. Both provide an equitable environment for the practice of a sport. Within sport for the disabled competitors are classified by their body's degree of function, and therefore it is important that the classification process is robust and achieves equity across the Paralympic sporting practice, enabling athletes to compete on a 'level playing field':

> A basic goal of classification is to ensure that winning or losing an event depends on talent, training, skill, fitness, and motivation rather than unevenness among competitors on disability-related variables (e.g., spasticity, paralysis, absence of limb segments).
>
> (Sherrill 1999: 210)

In order to highlight many of the issues surrounding classification as a mode of governance, I turn to an account of my own classification done on the eve of my first Paralympic experience.

The classification of a body

Seoul – September 1988

After two days of travelling and very little sleep I am still unable to rest. The weather outside is very humid and the waiting area is far too small and cramped. To make matters worse there is limited seating. The nature of my impairment (mild cerebral palsy) means that I have suffered less from the travel than some of my fellow participants. Many athletes that use wheelchairs for mobility were confined to their seats for over fifteen hours. I should be delighted to be in Asia for the first time. The Paralympic Games in Seoul Korea have been the focus of my attention – sporting and otherwise – for the last three years. In order to get clearance to compete in Seoul

I am waiting in no-man's-land at the edge of the Paralympic village where I must go through the process of classification. Several weeks from now I will pit my wits (body and soul) against the best athletes in the world that are classified as cerebral palsy seven (CP 7). This is the presumed outcome of the classification process as I have been competing within the category for the past three years and my body is a textbook example of hemiplegia, the impairment that is at the heart of CP 7. In spite of this I must wait my turn to go through the classification drills. It is the waiting and uncertainty that bother me with regards to classification. From time to time the classification process, has been engaged in too close to my races, but at least this time we are a couple of weeks away from my first competition.

Being pigeon-holed as a particular type of 'body' is an odd experience. It determines many things within sport for the disabled – for example, with whom I am allocated a shared room within the athletes village, and whether or not I am considered an elite athlete.[2] Why should the impaired body that I possess influence living arrangements and my status as an athlete? I am well trained, regularly running 100 miles a week. Can others not see beyond my CP and see that I am as committed as any middle- or long-distance runner, regardless of my impaired state?

Here we go! It is my turn next after four hours in this sterile room. The wait is over. My classification begins. To date I have undergone the process of classification three times. It is an alienating experience, as each time a different team of individuals determines whether your body fits into the textbook of carnal typology that is acceptable to those who govern the particular element of Paralympic sport that the athletes wish to be a part.

My body is poked and prodded. It is measured. I am asked to walk, run and jump in a room that is really not suitable for any physical activity whatsoever. Too small to build up a head of steam while running, and lacking ventilation so that I am grateful that I cannot run. This is unfortunate, because my impairment means that I have trouble controlling my muscles and stopping is as tricky as starting to run. This is a result of spasticity brought on by my cerebral palsy. In essence I am a 'spaz', as the public might refer to my physical state.

The classifiers see me as a difficult character. On several occasions I am told to simply 'do as they ask' and not to bother them with 'trivial' questions. What strikes me as odd is how questions regarding the medical state of my body can be seen as trivial in light of the fact that the process of classification will enable me to compete it the Paralympic Games. Later, in the Paralympic village, I hear stories of athletes who try to cheat the system. That is, they try to make their bodies appear more impaired than they actually are so that they are classed with a more impaired group. The result of such fraudulent activity means that they will have a better chance of winning, but it most certainly is antithetical to the ethics of the practice communitas.

The team of classifiers look like they have been working all night long, and I wonder whether this will lead to an inaccurate diagnosis. Will any of the athletes I race against have beaten the system? It seems robust, but rumours of cheating abound. Each team comprises a medical doctor, a physiotherapist and a sports technical expert.[3] One assumes the technical expert would be different if I had been attempting to compete in swimming rather than athletics. It transpires that the sport technical person on the classification team is normally someone trained in physical education or kinesiology and therefore has an understanding of 'movement and sport' in a general sense. None of these individuals are particularly friendly, in part due to the drawn out nature of the process, but they also appear to have treated me as a specimen pickled in formaldehyde and placed on a shelf in a biology classroom. My body has been processed – classified – as an object of medical science where my disembodied identity does not seem matter.

I was 'successful' in classification, as expected. I will be competing in the CP 7 class. Unsurprisingly it turns out my roommate is also a CP 7 athlete, though while my impairment is congenital his is the result of a head injury. Other than the degree of cerebral palsy and the spasticity it creates when fatigued (a regular occurrence for athletes with CP), we have little in common. I am concerned as to whether I will be able to 'live' with someone I have little in common with, other than an impaired embodiment, for the next three-and-a-half weeks. How will these living arrangements impact upon my performances on the track? Is the process of classification simply a way of controlling the bodies that contest the Paralympic Games?

Key to the political debate regarding classification is the historical development of sport for the disabled (Steadward 1996; Vanlandewijck and Chappel 1996; Daly and Vanlandewijck 1999) that segments a small population into sometimes even non-existent competition classes. The charitable ethos of the IOSDs (see Jones and Howe 2005) has led the Paralympic Movement to celebrate participation over performance for much of its history. Since the first codification of rules detailing the practice of sport for the disabled in 1972 (see Chapter 2) there has been a slow move toward high-performance sport, and from the mid-1980s, with three distinct impairment groups involved, the simplification of classification within the sports has become politically imperative. As a result, the classification system developed by the IOSDs is considered incompatible with high-performance sport by most within the IPC (Howe and Jones 2006).

Controlling Paralympic bodies

Processes of classification within sport for the disabled make distinctions between the physical potential of athletes and attempt to achieve an equitable environment whereby, after competition, the successful athletes in each class will have an equal chance of accumulating physical capital (Jones and Howe

2005). In reality, however, there are a number of factors that impact upon the accumulation of capital (both physical and cultural) in various classifications. The first factor is the number of athletes within a particular event. If there are only a handful, then the amount of capital that can be accumulated in most cases is limited. In some classes there may only be six athletes from four countries (the IPC minimum for eligible events), which means winners are less likely to receive the same kudos as an athlete who defeats twenty athletes. Another important factor in terms of whether winners ultimately gain capital from their involvement in sport is the nature and degree of their impairment. A component of the culture of elite sport for the disabled is a hierarchy of 'acceptable' impairment (Sherrill and Williams 1996; Schell and Rodriguez 2001), which is directly linked to the classification of athletes.

The Paralympic Games' second largest sport (in terms of the number of competitors) is swimming, and has, in conjunction with the IPC, developed a sport specific classification system. An integrated functional classification system that combined athletes who 'traditionally' were under the care and classification of separate IOSDs has been part of the organisation of IPC international swimming competitions since 1989 (Wu and Williams 1999). This system allows for the combining of physical[4] impairment groups into ten classes so that they can compete together. The reduction in the number of classes is believed to have a number of benefits: 'Not only has the number of classes been reduced from 31 to 10, there has been a reduction in the cancellation of events and the number of races in which swimmers from several classes take part' (Wu and Williams 1999: 263). The latter point is crucial. The previous disability-specific classification systems were hierarchical, so that if two events needed to be combined then the athletes from the less impaired class were bound to dominate. By reducing the number of classes, the likelihood of combinations has also been removed; however, it also means that there is great variation in ability within each class.

The practice community reflected in the IOSDs (see Howe and Jones 2006) established a system where athletes with a disability were able to enjoy equitable sporting competition. Many of the first officials of the IPC had previously held posts within these founding federations. Initially this allowed for acceptance of the IOSD's classification systems in the early days of the IPC. One of the legacies of this heritage is a complex classification system that many in the IPC now regard as cumbersome, as logistically problematic and as a potential threat to the marketability of the Games (see Chapter 5).

> One of the major difficulties in developing any classification system ... is handling the assumption that all individuals in the same category demonstrate a similar performance standard. Decreasing the number of classes in a system increases the number of swimmers in each class. This is desirable when the goal is to increase the credibility of the whole swimming competition, but it is extremely problematic in single events because it increases the potential for differences between swimmers.
>
> (Wu and Williams 1999: 264)

The IPC swimming integrated functional classification system includes what is known as a 'bench test', where the swimmers' range of motion of their various joints, muscular strength and limb co-ordination are determined on a physio-therapy bench (Dummer 1999). A swimming test then shows the athlete's ability to maintain horizontal body position and perform various technical skills that are necessary in competitive swimming, such as starts, strokes and turns. Points are awarded for both the bench test and the swimming test, and athletes are classified in three ways depending on the event in which they wish to compete: S class for freestyle, backstroke and butterfly; SB for breaststroke; and SM for individual medley.

Advocates of the integrated functional classification system currently in place in IPC swimming believe that the statistics show that competition is relatively fair although '[b]ecause sport performance is dynamic, absolute criteria for fairness cannot be based on competitive results alone' (Daly and Vanlandewijck 1999: 273). The integrated functional classification system does allow for more spectac-ular competition, by creating fewer classes and less confusion among the public and sponsors alike. Viable races are also produced by the system, because they consistently involve a sufficient number of competitors and are therefore unlikely to be cancelled or haphazardly combined at the last minute. This said, most stat-istics used for this evaluation are based on competitive results, so last-minute event cancellation would not be evident in the data (Daly and Vanlandewijck 1999). The elimination of over 21 classes through this integrated classification system means that it serves the aims of the IPC to simplify and speed up events, but I contend that it does not necessarily serve the best interests of the practice community (Morgan 1994a). In contrast, the impairment-specific functional clas-sification system adopted in athletics may better serve the practice communitas, since each class is not as diverse in terms of varied levels of ability.

The acceptance of an integrated functional classification system in swimming, where ability rather than disability was the focus, and the resulting elimination of a complex system of impairment-specific classification systems made this an agenda item at all the IPCAC meetings I attended. The IPCAC was (and I believe still is) under pressure from the IPC to develop an integrated functional classification system that is equivalent to that for swimming. Because the IPCAC had a representative from each IOSD on the committee, there was an impasse regarding discussions surrounding classification. Each IOSD representative essen-tially believed in the validity of his or her own classification system, and was willing to give little ground. This situation existed until 2006, when representa-tion from all the IOSDs was no longer part of the IPCAC committee structure.

It is understandable that the IOSDs' representatives were concerned that their athletes should not be disadvantaged by a new classification system. As I commented in my field notes after a meeting:

It seems ridiculous that one item on an agenda seven items long can take up so much time. In this case seventy-five percent of the meeting. Classifi-cation always seems to be the sticky wicket. Discussion of classification, while dominating proceedings, is worrying because it means that the various IOSDs are not consulting their athletes or their classification teams when important discussions are being debated. This important element of sport for the disabled needs to find resolutions within the IOSD before it can be resolved at the level of the IPC. We are after all talking about individuals whose quality of life will be radically affected if their class folds or is merged with another. In a world where team selection is often based upon who will bring home a medal, classification does matter but the system should not be squeezed to the point where the tail is wagging the dog. At the minute the debates about classification within IPC athletes suggest that athletes really do not matter.

This recap from a particularly heated meeting of the IPCAC highlights a number of issues that are central to the politics surrounding sport for the disabled. First of all there is the relationship between the IPC and the IOSDs, which is often tense at best because the former has done little to develop sporting talent at the grass-roots level. The IOSDs feel they have the best interests of their athletes as their central concerns. On another level, the IOSDs seldom consult their athlete membership as to how the federation should be organised and run. Many athletes are keen to embrace the aims and goals of the IPC, yet in committee meetings IOSD representatives are often unwilling to acknowledge this. There is a lack of communication between athletes and administrators, who either work on behalf of the IPC or IOSDs, which in the political environment of the Paralympic Movement also has a huge cultural component. While there are few non-Western representatives on IPC committees, the establishment of geographic regions of the IPC may be a step in the right direction. The IPC has divided the world into five regions (Africa, the Americas, Asia, Europe and Oceania). These regions are to help augment the political influence of the IPC, but tension has begun to develop concerning accurate regional representation on all central IPC committees that have traditionally been Eurocentric.

The establishment of better regional representation does not stop the battle for classification between the IOSDs and the IPC. Since 2002, the IPCAC has taken control of classification at all its major events. During the 1990s the IOSDs had classification teams present at every major IPC event to ensure that their federation's rules were properly applied. Now, in the case of athletics, the IPC interprets the rules of the IOSDs. Interpretation of the rules allows the IPC to classify athletes in a different manner from that of the IOSD. I have known athletes to be used as pawns in this political battle, with the IPC and the IOSD giving the same body a different classification. This shows that the systems of classification need to be both better policed (with the athletes' interest at heart) and more robust. In order to situate this analysis in the cultural environment surrounding the Paralympic sport, it is important now to turn to a discussion of the culture of IPC athletics and the role it plays within the classification process.

Classification in IPC athletics

Despite the adoption of an integrated functional classification system within swimming, political pressure from the IOSDs and disagreements within the sport, the disability-specific classification systems have been retained in the sport of athletics. The habitus of the sport of Paralympic athletics means that the IOSDs developed systems that provide an equitable playing field on which athletes within a disability group can compete against one another. The federations have attempted to structure competition so that only similarly affected athletes compete against one another – an amputee athlete does not compete against an athlete with cerebral palsy, for example. They use functionally specific guidelines to place the athlete in a suitable competitive class. The process of classification is normally undertaken when individuals first become involved in sport for the disabled, and often confirmed when they attend their first major international competition such as the Paralympic Games. Given the number and complexity of the classification systems within each disability group, the organisation of competitions is logistically complicated. There were fifteen 100 m final races[5] for men and eleven for women in the sport of athletics in the 2000 Paralympic Games, compared with one final race per sex for the 100 m at the Olympic Games.

The many classes eligible for participation in the Paralympics programme led the IPC to implement a rule in 1992 that required an event to have at least six competitors from four nations to make it viable within the Games. While such a rule would be unlikely to have significance in mainstream sport, it has had a profound impact on the viability of some sports within the Paralympic programme. Within athletics, this rule ignited the debate about the type of classification system to be used in the sport. Disagreement in athletics over the equity of different systems of classification and the best way to achieve fairness in competition was central to this debate. To date the debate has resulted in a stalemate, and the disability-specific classification system within athletics continues to be used. This has meant that many athletic events for the more severely impaired and women have been cancelled or combined in recent years on IPC athletics programmes. Due to the importance placed upon equitable competition, the disability-specific classification systems may create competitive pools that produce insufficient numbers of competitors to meet the IPC regulations for viable competition. In addition, the IPC Athletics Committee has recently ruled that an event must have at least ten athletes on its official ranking list for it to be considered for the Paralympic or World Championship programmes. Events with a small number of competitors have been placed under considerable strain as a result. The problem of low numbers of competitors is exacerbated by the onset of injury in an already small number of athletes (Howe 2004a, 2006a). The practice communitas is being compelled by the IPC to adhere to a policy that in no way resembles the key principle of Paralympism: the empowerment of athletes with a disability.

The specification of a minimum numbers of athletes within an event has significantly influenced the organisation of Paralympic athletics. The cancellation of an event altogether or, in some cases, the movement of competitors to a less impaired class in order to make the event viable has an impact on future programmes. A competitor who is moved to a less impaired class is not competing on a level playing field and is unlikely to win. Although winning is not central to Paralympism as formulated by the IPC, it is a major consideration for National Paralympic Committees when making team selections. National Paralympic Committees emphasise winning since they receive greater publicity and increased funding based upon their position in the medal table. Individual nations are therefore not concerned whether events are removed from the programme unless they have athletes that were potential medallists. Events disappear from the Paralympic programme and from future programmes because of the apparent disinterest by those in the relevant classification grouping, when in fact it is not solely athletes making the decision but their National Paralympic Committee in conjunction with the IPC.

There are several ways that the sport of athletics has tried to rectify this issue of a low number of entries within constituent events in the sport. For example, IPC athletics has considered combining wheelchair classes in track events. Both the Cerebral Palsy-International Sport and Recreation Association (CP-ISRA) and the International Wheelchair and Amputee Sport Association (IWAS) have athletes who compete from a sitting position in a wheelchair. At the current time, elite male wheelchair CP-ISRA athletes are in limited supply. Although the classes would meet the IPC criteria of six athletes from four countries for Paralympic eligibility, the IPC Athletics Committee has suggested that they would not be competitive enough. Consequently, it has removed the last remaining men's cerebral palsy wheelchair classes from the Paralympic programme. In a bid to improve the quality of racing and to ensure that a small number of competitors does not become an issue in the future for the small number of CP-ISRA male athletes, the IPC Athletics Committee has combined two impairment classifications of male wheelchair racers. Rather than trying to establish an equitable system where existing classes from both federations are the starting point for a new system, administrators have merged classes of cerebral palsy athletes into the IWAS classification system. The IPC wanted to establish an official rule for a combined system for athletics competitors in wheelchairs before the 2006 World Championships after testing it at the 2002 World Championships and the 2004 Paralympic Games. While such a rule has not been formalised in practice it was used in 2006 at the World Championships, and it is just a matter of time before it is made official, with little resistance in spite of the problems with establishing a consensus about what is fair for all competitors. In addition, from 2006 the practice communitas (IOSDs) no longer has membership in the IPC Athletics Committee.

Many difficulties exist in attempting to combine all athletic competitors in wheelchairs. For example, the location of the lesion on the spine influences the degree of power that can be generated by those with a spinal injury impairment. Meanwhile, athletes with cerebral palsy who race in a wheelchair cope with issues of motor control (Richter 1999). Combining all users of wheelchairs in athletics is problematic, as it becomes an issue of giving points to athletes involved in the classification process based on two distinct components; power and control. In fact, no point system for the ratio between power and control has yet been established as part of the IWAS classification system. Since power and control are distinct elements in managing embodied performance, it would be inappropriate for those involved in classification of wheelchair track athletes not to establish a relationship between these two components of movement. Class 3 and 4 cerebral palsy athletes are currently placed in Classes 2 and 3 of the IWAS system because world-best performances for these athletes were similar to average performances in their respective IWAS class.

During the 2002 IPC World Championships, three male athletes with cerebral palsy were competitive enough to qualify in their new class. All were world-record holding athletes in their respective cerebral palsy classes, but struggled to get out of their heats when competing against their 'equals' from the IWAS. So the question remains, how can this system be considered equitable when it collapses two distinct forms of impairment into one class and those with one form consistently achieve superior competitive results across the board? Only two men made the grade for the 2004 Athens Paralympics while the other retired, disenchanted with the sport. Using performance as a premise for classification in the context of sport for the disabled appears to contradict the principle of equity on which systems of classification should be based (Richter 1999). Fortunately, CP-ISRA women's wheelchair events are still a viable part of the Paralympic programme.[6] At other IPC international events, the combining of the male wheelchair classes has brought about the demise of elite male wheelchair racing for athletes with cerebral palsy, even though it continues to attract high-level performances at the CP-ISRA World Championships.

In contrast to track events, IPC athletics has adopted a distinct approach to organising field events when there are insufficient competitors in one class to stage a viable competition. Classes are combined across the IOSD system using decathlon-style tables, facilitating viable competition from low athlete numbers across numerous classes (see Chapter 3). Each individual sporting performance is assigned points based on existing tables established for each class. The winner is determined not by the furthest distance thrown or length/height of jump, but by the number of points each effort is worth. In principle this system of tables could be used in track events, but the nature of athletics means that it has a first-past-the-post approach to competition. In track events the winner is selected by running in direct competition with other athletes over standardised distances, whereas in the field competitors are arguably competing against themselves. It could be argued that tactics in the high jump, which is a Paralympic event for the visually impaired and amputee competitors, come into play in the count-back rituals – where the athlete who has missed the least attempts has an advantage. Other than in this situation, field events require competition against oneself as the format is not head-to-head. The first-past-the-post principle means that carte blanche adoption of tables for track events as well as the field would be considered undesirable by the IPC since it would 'ruin' the spectacle. Many spectators would be disappointed after watching a nail-biting finish to a race only to find out that the athlete in fifth place actually won, as has occurred in swimming events within recent Commonwealth Games.

Swimmers in the Commonwealth Games competed against the best performances in their class, and not necessarily other competitors. As a result, the winner was chosen not as a result of the fastest overall time but rather by the best result in comparison to their class record. This means the swimmer that wins may not be the fastest in the pool, which impacts on the spectacle of any given race. In fairness to those who organised the elite athletes with a disability events at these Games, a limited number of eligible athletes in any one class meant that events needed to be combined, to fill every lane in the pool with athletes from different countries. The most equitable way of holding such a race was to have each athlete compete against their class's world-record performance.

Classifier as gatekeeper

Classifiers working within the Paralympic Movement are more often then not 'able'. The sport of athletics appears to be 'policed' by the 'able', or AB as the other athletes refer to them. As a result, individuals who work on classification teams may be seen as agents of social control (Wu *et al.* 2000). In recent years the financial benefits associated with the Paralympic Games have increased. This, I would argue, is a direct reason for changes to the classification process and regulation within the Movement. Changes to classification systems have been about packaging the most attractive and commercially viable product that will be sold to the highest bidder. By transforming classification where an equitable chance of achieving success is lost for the price of media interest, the practice communitas is altered.

The practice communitas in sport for the disabled is made up of both primary and secondary agents (Howe and Jones 2006). Athletes are primary agents because, in a traditional view of sporting practice, they are considered of greatest importance. In other words, they are the reason for a sport. Secondary agents, on the other hand, consist of medical staff, coaches, game officials, volunteer administrators, spectators and journalists who organise, regulate and maintain sporting practice. Many secondary agents have been involved with the practice communitas and then have moved into leading roles within the IPC, which, as an institution, is still in its infancy. The flexible boundaries between institution and the practice communitas make it difficult to establish who is sincerely concerned with the cultural practice of high-performance sport for the disabled.

As a result, the distinction between primary and secondary agents within practice communities is important, but it can be difficult to sustain and, moreover, fails to adequately address the heterogeneous nature of these groups. An athlete, for example, may have been born with a disability or may have acquired it from some form of trauma later in life. Athletes can also be distinguished as members of sub-groupings by their race, ethnicity, class and gender, both inside and outside of a given practice communitas, and their identity is not simply tied to their impairment. In addition, athletes may vary in the degree to which they value internal and external goods. As primary agents within the practice communitas, athletes are interested in the internal goods of the their chosen sport (Morgan 1994a). Internal goods are peculiar to the practice, such as the skills required to perform in a given sport such as athletics. Athletes may, however, become tempted by the external goods or economic capital acquired by institutions such as the IPC, and begin to feel that their labours need rewarding.

The shift in focus from internal goods to external goods is something that can also readily befall secondary agents, particularly those eager to gain or establish their position within the structure of the IPC. Secondary agents are primarily able-bodied persons who may have been involved in sport themselves, but usually not in sport for the disabled. Able-bodied sports facilitators may be aware of the internal goods of a particular sport, but their experience is different from that of disabled athletes because they are not disabled themselves. The able-bodied can also take it upon themselves to highlight the problems with the process of classification, as the scandal described below attests.

Scandal over INAS-FID classification

Athletes with intellectual disabilities had first been involved in the Paralympic Games in Atlanta in 1996. In 1994, a small number had been eligible to compete in demonstration events at the IPC World Athletic Championships. Many athletes from other disability federations were unhappy with athletes from the INAS-FID being included, suggesting that they belong in the Special Olympics (BBC 1994). Unlike the other IOSDs, the classification system of the INAS-FID is based upon the measurement of Intelligent Quotient (IQ). Athletes are required to have an IQ of less than 75 to be eligible for competition. At the Games in Atlanta, I wrote in my notebook:

> The classification process for intellectually disabled athletes seems a bit odd. Talking to a few of them in the village it seems that for most they 'suffer' from different socialisation than most of the other athletes. There may be a case for including them in the Games because they seem to lack an ability to focus on anything for an extended period of time. It is unfortunate but how do you make a robust classification system that will police those who are eligible? Is IQ not a rather culturally specific test? If so, how do you know where people are cheating?

In Sydney, a journalist from Spain reported in the magazine *Capital* on 21 November 2000 that he and ten of the twelve-member Gold Medal basketball squad had not been eligible to compete. It was found that one-third of the INAS-FID athletes had been correctly classified (Cashman 2006: 268). The

IPC has suspended the federation until it produces verifiable classification tests. INAS-FID athletes missed the Athens Games and, at the time of going to press, are considered ineligible to compete in the Games of 2008. This scandal has acted as a wake-up call for the IPC, and is likely to be one of the primary motivations for the establishment of the code for classification that was highlighted above.

Decisions regarding the viability of sports classification systems and competition may not necessarily be congruent with decisions about the interests of athletes with a disability The provision of competitive categories that maximise participation may satisfy the inclusive aims of the IOSDs, but might undermine the IPC's desire to provide contests for highly motivated and skilled elite athletes. In addition, the talent pool may be spread too thinly across too many events. With heterogeneity so evident within the practice communitas, there appears to be a need for open and frank discussions in order to establish the best way forward. The danger is that the IPC is in such a powerful position, with support from many quarters, including the IOC, that the IOSDs may have missed an important opportunity to shape sport for the disabled in an athlete-friendly manner.

Summary

Within the body culture of which the practice of athletics is a part, the need to develop an equitable system of classification is politically problematic. It is not surprising, therefore, that the politics of disability is concerned that the body is the obstacle for inclusion into society.

The classification of my body highlighted above occurred directly after the Olympic Games, in Seoul. If my body were classified today, the result would be the same. My classification has not changed, but the landscape of sport for the disabled has. The governance of sport for the disabled, in part through the implementation of various classification systems, has allowed both the IPC and at various times the IOSDs to control the political landscape. Importantly, the structure of classification allows for the control of impaired bodies. Classification ultimately takes autonomy away from the athletes. This is no different from mainstream sport, except that the IPC and the IOSDs trade on the fact that they are working on behalf of the athletes. A close examination of the politics associated with classification suggests this is not the case, and the IPC clearly has more pressing matters on its agenda. Under the supervision of the IPC there has been a move toward the commercialisation of sport for the disabled that has been managed in partnership with increased media coverage of flagship events (Schantz and Gilbert 2001; Schell and Rodriguez 2001; Smith and Thomas 2005) – an issue to which I turn in the next chapter.

5   Mediated Paralympic culture

Anyone that has followed the developments in the Paralympic Movement since the mid-1980s will be aware of the transformation in the commercial viability of the IPC. In 1984 the Movement was unable to stage the entire Games in the same nation as that year's Olympics (United States of America), whereas today the regular reference in the same breath to the Olympics and the Paralympics is a major advance. This has occurred in part because of the political battles that have been waged between the IPC and IOSDs, highlighted in the last few chapters of this monograph. In part changes in attitude are the result of increased media attention given to the Paralympic Movement, which has had an impact on the transformation of institutional structures such as classification. This chapter will argue that such attention has come at a price.

Links between the Olympic and Paralympic Movements are more explicit than ever. The process of a city bidding to be the host of the Olympic Games must now include a proposal for how the Paralympics will be managed. Explicit financial support from the Olympic Movement has been almost non-existent, at least until the 2004 Games in Athens, but the more wholesome image of the Paralympics certainly benefits the Olympics by association (Balding 2004). However, some have suggested that this is a very unequal relationship. Recently there has been criticism regarding the unequal treatment of the Paralympics in relation to the Olympics. Goggin and Newell (2000) have argued that the Paralympics in Sydney were not treated as positively as the Olympics. 'While cities compete aggressively for the right to host an Olympic Games, they inherit the Paralympic Games as an obligation' (Cashman 2006: 247). Fears of financial sustainability, which were of concern to Ludwig Guttmann (Goodman 1986; Scruton 1998), seem to be a thing of the past, but the question that concerns us here is whether the IPC, in its new commercially more comfortable situation, can be true to its heritage. This means explicitly working towards providing equal opportunities for all impairment groups in equitable sporting competition at the high-performance end of the sport for the disabled spectrum.

As the last chapter highlighted, classification is a perennial political issue. Since 2006 the IPC Classification Committee has been pushing ahead with the development of a code for classification so that all IPC sports follow the same guidelines in the process of determining the eligibility of athletes. The IPC has, as recently as spring 2007, been soliciting opinions from a range of individuals with a concern for equity within the process in order to reshape the complex disability-specific classification system. According to Steadward (1996: 36), 'the potential benefit of decreasing classes by using a functional integrated classification system is that it may simplify the integration into the rest of the sports world'. The adoption of a code of practice for classification to which all IPC sports must adhere is a sign of the new professionalism of the Paralympic Movement, where there is a desire for all concerned to be dealing with classification in the same manner.

Under the supervision of the IPC there has been a move toward the commercialisation of sport for the disabled that has been managed in partnership with increased media coverage of flagship events (Schantz and Gilbert 2001; Schell and Rodriguez 2001; Smith and Thomas 2005). Prior to the establishment of the IPC classification code, streamlining of competitive programmes in sports such as athletics was rather ad hoc. In Chapter 4 I highlighted how the sport of athletics requires ten athletes to be on a ranking list in order for an event to run in the Paralympic programme. This has put increasing pressure on the classification system in athletics. A reduction in the number of classes competing means that the athletics programme is streamlined, but ultimately that there may be no sporting provision for certain impairment types creating an inequality of opportunity. Such a move is incompatible with the ethos of Paralympism (see Chapter 2), but ultimately leads to an increase in the number of viable events at major championships (Vanlandewijck and Chappel 1996: 70–71). As such, the resulting programme of events is more attractive to the mainstream media and ultimately helps attract sponsorship.

Attracting sponsors

Creating interest in sponsorship opportunities for the Paralympic Movement has been a difficult task. During the lead-up to the 1996 Games in Atlanta, where there were separate organising committees for the Olympics and the Paralympics, it was felt that sponsorship could be secured from businesses tailored to the large American disabled communitas. However, only Atlanta-based soft drinks manufacturer Coca Cola came forward to supply beverages to the Paralympic Games, although it gave no other financial support (BBC 1994). The assumption that the disabled communitas would support this or any other Paralympic Games was a mistake. A year before the 2000 Games in Sydney, the IPC was struggling to get financial support. Optimé International, then working on marketing for the IPC, highlighted the plight of attracting sponsorship in a piece that ran in a Canadian newspaper entitled 'Faster, Higher, Poorer' (Cole 1999). This piece of publicity was timely. The article hit the press just as the IPC was due to open its first permanent headquarters in Bonn, Germany – an event that was held in conjunction with a conference, a large part of which focused upon issues related to classification and how the streamlining of the systems used could improve the commercialism and profitability of the IPC. The running of an international sporting federation is an expensive undertaking, and the IPC was keen to gain corporate support, much like the Olympic Movement has done.

In the lead-up to the 2000 Games, those in the corridors of power at the IPC had concerns regarding the lack of corporate sponsorship for the Movement. The then President, Dr Bob Steadward, suggested 'we know that the severity of disability can be unsettling for some people, because it's a reminder, a reality check, of how fragile the human body is. Some companies, I'm sure, fear that image' (Cole 1999). This tactic did not seem to pay many dividends. It was not until the Paralympic Movement forged closer links with the Olympic Movement that large corporate sponsors became interested. Benefits of the agreement between the two organisations included long-term financial support, access to high-quality facilities in which to hold the Paralympics, and countless other commercial bonuses. The first agreement between the IOC and IPC was signed in 2001 to formalise these closer ties. In 2003 this agreement was amended to transfer 'broadcasting and marketing responsibilities of the 2008, 2010, and 2012 Paralympic Games to the Organizing Committee of these Olympic and Paralympic Games' (IPC 2003a: 1).

These agreements will certainly ease financial concerns for the IPC; they will also put financial pressure on the practice community regarding the need to streamline classification (Howe and Jones 2006). It is important, therefore, to characterise elite disabled athletes as actors central to the Paralympic Movement. The conceptualisation of the practice community, as articulated by Morgan (1994a, 2002), allows for the distinction between the institution (in this case the IPC) and the practice community (which comprises those who are actively involved with the practice, i.e. athletes, coaches and officials of the IOSDs). The IOC requires that the Paralympic Games be restricted in size to 4000 athletes, which will benefit the IPC's commercial agenda because this size limitation will make the Paralympics a more manageable product to market. The marketing of the Olympics and Paralympics as a single entity has undermined the IPC's autonomy to use the Paralympic Games to educate the public about athletes with a disability. The erosion of this educational imperative is problematic, because one of the IPC's explicit aims is the effective and efficient promotion of elite sport for the disabled. Such erosion goes against the tenets of Paralympism (see Chapter 2), and as a result may not be in the best interest of the athletes.

As the IPC becomes increasing commercialised, there is an imperative for the athletes, coaches and officials to become more professional in the manner in which they engage in the practice of Paralympic sport. The IPC headquarters in Bonn has a ever-growing full-time staff that look after not only the practical side of sports but also issues related to development, finance, fundraising and sponsorship, as well as marketing and communication.[1] Multinational sponsors such as VISA and Samsung have invested considerable amounts of money in the IPC, and Otto Bock HealthCare has provided money and services to users of wheelchairs and prosthetic limbs during the Games. Whether these large

Table 5.1 Media details since 1988

	Athletes	Number of nations	Number of sports	Tickets sold	Television rights – fees	Accredited media
1988 Seoul	3053	62	17	Nil		1672
1992 Barcelona	3020	82	15	Nil		1499
1996 Atlanta	3310	103	17	388 373	$500 000	2088
2000 Sydney	3843	122	18	1 160 000	$4 200 000	2440
2004 Athens	3837	136	19	800 000		3000

Source: Cashman 2006: 251.

sponsors are a result of the close relationship between the IPC and IOC is unclear, although links with its mainstream brethren cannot have hindered the process of commercialisation.

Table 5.1 highlights a dramatic increase in media interest in the Paralympic Games. The number of accredited media has almost doubled since the 1988 Games. As a result, the public will be learning more about the Paralympic Movement with every passing Paralympiad. The Sydney 2000 Paralympics made a profit of $31.2 million (Cashman 2006: 258). The commercial prospects for those hosting the Paralympics has improved, although it is not the as profitable as the Olympic Games.

It might be assumed that attention which is an accurate reflection of Paralympic culture is the aim of interested media exposure. However, an interesting by-product of an increasingly commercial IPC has been an inaccurate representation of Paralympic culture in the media. Whether an inaccurate representation of Paralympians is intentional or not, it does little to lessen the social burden of disability on Paralympic athletes and as such is an important issue to which chapter will now turn.

Paralympic (sub)culture

So influential is the role played by the those constructing images of the Paralympic Movement that it is often portrayed as a (sub)culture of the mainstream sport culture with elements of sporting cultures of the amateur age – purity, innocence and integrity. As the IPC has 'progressed' towards full commercialism these ideals have been, in reality, if not lost then increasingly obscured from view. In essence, print-media journalists and other forms of media more generally have framed Paralympic sport as a (sub)culture, establishing boundaries around it but seldom exploring what in fact makes it culturally distinctive.

To date, the social scientific research on the media and elite disabled athletes has been primarily concerned with issues of representation (Schantz and Gilbert 2001; Schnell and Rodriguez 2001; Smith and Thomas 2005) that have been both static and disembodied. This work, while not explicitly suggesting sport for the disabled is a subculture, does imply that this sporting environment is distinctive. Following Jenks (2005), the marginal is romanticised in postmodern cultural politics – an arena in which research on media representation of Paralympic Sport can be situated. Therefore, for the purpose of this monograph a

> 'subculture' can be seen as ways of containment, as a kind of cognitive wrapping paper and string with which to bundle up clusters of deviance, criminality, ethnicity, poverty or just generations.
>
> (Jenks 2005: 144)

By extension, we can assume disability can be contained in this way. I now briefly turn to a brief discussion of Bourdieu's conceptualisation of habitus as it relates to sports journalism before I explicitly enter the field myself.

Habitus, sport and journalism

The conceptual understanding of habitus outlined by Pierre Bourdieu is useful in examining the cultural milieu surrounding the production of media texts. To Bourdieu, habitus informs action like grammar structures a language, which can allow for multiple forms of expression through the body – whether it is how the body moves or how it is covered (Bourdieu 1984). The habitus of the social agents involved in the production of the Paralympics, whether they are athletes, administrators or journalists recording the spectacle, is 'players' in a game actively working toward achieving a goal with acquired skills and competence but doing so within an established structure of rules which are only gradually transformed over time. Habitus predisposes action by agents, but does not reduce them to a position of complete subservience.

Bourdieu (1990a) explores the philosophy behind gymnastics, and from this it can be ascertained that other structured sporting activities are cultural products developed over a long period of time by those who are involved in their practice. The embodiment of these products is distinctive to the (sub)culture. In other words, for Bourdieu an agent's habitus is the embodied sediment of every encounter they have had with the social world. It can be used in the present to mould perception, thought and action to the extent that it has an important role to play in decisions that an agent might make in future encounters. In this sense actors (athletes, officials and journalists) can be seen not simply as following rules but also as bending them, much in the same way as the work of Merleau-Ponty (1962, 1965) highlights improvisation as being fundamental to an individual's disposition. Dispositions, or more generally forms of social competence, may be seen as a product of well-established social environments. While society may be seen as shaping agents, it needs individuals' improvisations from time to time if it is going to evolve. Therefore, in the post-industrial society in which we live, it is as important to see the body as being as much a product of the self as it is of society. It is the self that provides improvisation by drawing upon the sediment of previous social encounters.

The theory of practice developed by Bourdieu (1977, 1990a) identifies the nexus between the body and the social environment surrounding it. In a sporting context, then, the games metaphor that is employed by Bourdieu in both non-sporting and sporting contexts highlights the nexus between capital and field. The multiplication of players' disposition, their competence (habitus) and the resources at their disposal (capital) in relation to the social environment highlights the social actors' position in the world. In the particular environment that is elite sport, it is the embodied disposition or doxa that enables a social exploration of the distinctive character of sporting practice and body hexis that is the performative aspect of habitus. In a sense, embodied sporting practice is made up of the habitual disposition established through the training drills (as athlete, administrator or journalist) that might be part of a traditional training regime and the desire actually to play the game. Paralympic practice is therefore structured at a number of levels, with improvisation grounded in sediments of previous activities.

The structure of the Paralympic (sub)culture is also imposed in the form of rules and regulations that have been codified by sporting federations. Rules are imposed upon individuals who fall under the federation's authority including athletes, officials and journalists. The social environment of sport is determined by all three levels of structure, but still allows room for improvisation on the part of the participant. This field or network configuration (Bourdieu and Wacquant 1992: 97) therefore allows the social scientist to see beyond the body as object and allow for an appropriate conceptualisation within the sporting environment. Capital, on the other hand, allows for the exploration of the issues associated with assets, both economic and cultural, which a disposition may have in a particular social field (Bourdieu 1990b: 63).

The physical action of a participant within the Paralympic (sub)culture is strategic, and the better it is the more embodied cultural capital or physical capital a participant possesses (Wacquant 1995; Shilling 2003). For example, the qualities that are associated with sports journalism bodies such as the ability to forge an extensive network of contacts (informants), the ability to meet deadlines and the innate ability to know the 'real' story in amongst the rumble of continuous press releases are all part of a continuum of performance, and when a journalist achieves highly in any or all of these categories he or she will possess physical capital in the sporting environment (field) where those qualities are revered. The physical act of working with the social environment of the newsroom requires the journalist to perform (hexis) in the world of sports journalism. This structure of the social environment is a fundamental component of a journalist's habitus. This enables a journalist to work at times in an unreflective manner, which allows for access to sediments of past newsbeats to form the roots of new improvisations. A new member of the Paralympic (sub)culture may also see the importance of acquiring good skills as part and parcel of this social environment.

On the beat

In order to gain an understanding of Paralympic mediation and its role in creating a (sub)culture, I had to gain accreditation as a journalist at the Paralympic Games and be 'working' for a recognised publication or media outlet. Once this position was secured, approval also had to be obtained from the National Paralympic Committee. Accreditation was secured through the British Paralympic Association (BPA) for *Run, Throw and Jump*,[2] a weekly British track and field athletics publication. The BPA therefore was an important gatekeeper that controlled access for journalists based in Britain to the world of newswork (Allan 1999) at all IPC-sanctioned events. The editor at *Run, Throw and Jump* valued an appreciation of track and field athletics and an understanding of Paralympic sport over experience as a journalist.[3] Years reading *Run, Throw and Jump* facilitated an understanding of the type of prose that was expected from contributors. It is an enthusiasts' periodical that uses a simple narrative style. Appropriate use of the nomenclature of the sport of track and field athletics and a focus predominantly upon British successes was the brief for the beat. My aim was to provide detailed reports from 'trackside' so that their weekly coverage would be as 'culturally rich' as it would be for the Olympic Games.

Full media accreditation acted as a passport for Paralympic and Athens city public transport, as well as access to all areas associated with the Olympic venues (accept those reserved for VIPs, and the Paralympic village). In the media centre that was in the bowels of the Olympic stadium, the massive media machine that the Olympics creates was starkly visible. The media centre was so large it could have housed an indoor 200m athletics track. For the Paralympics (perhaps not surprisingly), the room was less than 20 per cent full. Due to the media centre's vastness, journalists were given a map that traced the quickest route to the key media points, including a ten-minute walk across the Olympic site to the International Broadcast Centre, in which the studios were located for the broadcast media. This media venue was even more barren. NBC, the American broadcaster that had the televisual rights to the Olympic Games, had pulled out all its 3500 staff after the closing ceremonies. One British journalist that had worked for a number of years on the Paralympic beat publicly criticised this move (Pryor 2004a). The fact that NBC did not even leave a shadow broadcast team was highlighted as a negative for the New York bidding team for the 2012 Games, because all the other nations that were bidding for the Games had maintained a degree of media presence during the Paralympics.

In spite of the empty space in both the media centre and the IBC, there were journalists of every form covering the Paralympic Games, many of whom had also worked at the Olympics three weeks earlier. The British Broadcasting Corporation (BBC) for the Athens Games had doubled the amount of coverage it had shown in Australia four years earlier, to an hour-and-a-half every evening. By the standards of the Paralympics this is a high level of coverage, but it falls well short of the coverage given by the same broadcaster to the Olympic

Games. Daily newspapers such as *The Times*, the *Daily Telegraph* and the *Daily Mail* all had print journalists present on the Paralympic beat.

The media centre under the Olympic stadium was to be the hub of my news-work for the ten days of the Paralympic athletics programme. Bearing this in mind, two things in particular stood out about the media centre other than the vastness of the complex. Both issues related to the inaccessibility of the environment. When holding a sporting event for athletes with a disability, ease of access for those with mobility impairment should be well organised. It was not. There was only one lift down to the heart of the media centre, and this lift only had room for one wheelchair. During the Paralympic Games it could be assumed that the whole Olympic site would be accessible, and the fact that the lift was small made an explicit statement that disabled people were not expected to be members of the media. For those who did gain access to the media centre, the area was full of other mobility pitfalls. Thousands of miles of electrical and fibre-optic cable were used to link up the stadium to the outside world. In the media centre most of this was on the floor, and though it was covered by metal protectors these were several inches wide and several inches high. As a result, these cable covers could be insurmountable barriers to a wheelchair user or an individual with a visual impairment. It would have been relatively simple to run the miles of cables under the floor – after all, the media centre was purpose-built – and have the cable required for the various workstations come up under each table. To add insult to injury, there was simply no attempt made to provide ramps over the cable covers. In interview, one of the heads of the media centre that was working on behalf of the IPC made it was clear that provision for the mobility-impaired journalist was not considered a priority.

> To my knowledge there are not any journalists here who have mobility issues. If we had been informed that there were a large number of disabled journalists we could have given them their own space.

This statement illustrates that some officials have limited understanding of the issues at the heart of the ideology of Paralympism. In fact, the number of disabled journalists was minimal. Over 95 per cent of the journalists in both the media centre and the IBC were able-bodied.

Inside the newsroom

Whether or not there should be a greater number of journalists with a disability working at the Paralympic Games is a contentious issue. Broadcasters and print publications at the Paralympic Games did not more readily use disabled journalists, and there seemed to be little concern about this imbalance. One able-bodied journalist for a British Sunday paper remarked

> Why should there be lots of journalists with disabilities here? Should we limit their opportunity to disabled events? Journalism is a competitive work

environment and only the best individuals should be covering a quality event like the Paralympic Games.

This statement suggests the field of journalism is not welcoming of principles such as positive discrimination. Perhaps because few impaired journalists were present in Athens, there was a distinctive element of the culture of the Paralympic beat that focuses on 'triumph over adversary', albeit from an able-bodied perspective. The employment of more journalists who understand the culture of sport for the disabled first-hand might in time redress this balance. Disabled individuals as overachievers are emphasised in most reporting. For example the journalists in Athens, as well as the IPC and their national affiliates, were invited to vote for recipients of the Whang Youn Dai *Overcome* Prize for the athlete that 'best represents the spirit of the Paralympic Games. This prize focuses on the determination of excellence of the mind, body and spirit in pursuit of sports *despite their adversities'*.[4]

One possible reason for the lack of disabled journalists is the speed of activity surrounding print-media production (Allan 1999; Lowe 1999). Most disabled people can work as quickly and efficiently as their able counterparts, however, the social stigma of disability implies a greater or lesser degree of inadequacy (Goffman 1963). At the Paralympics the speed of activity in the media centre was quite intense, especially when the journalists were closing in on their deadlines. Working for a weekly publication facilitated the ability to observe the mayhem without directly being a part of it. As the daily deadline approached, a sense of anxiety as to whether or not the journalist had the right quotes and the proper angle on each story ensued. These individuals constantly have their jobs in the balance. Journalists can lose their jobs if they fail to file regular copy that is deemed worthy of the audience of their publication.

Controlling the print media

At the Paralympics, the likelihood of not getting a story was eliminated by the way the beat was managed by both the IPC and its British affiliate, the BPA press office. Journalists huddled around the table used by the BPA press office in the media centre in order to obtain key pieces of information distributed by the office. Members of the BPA press office were crucial in shaping the culture of the Paralympic beat. They employed three able-bodied men (one of whom was a full-time employee) who resided in the media centre, and their responsibility was to collect quotes that would make for 'good ink' from the British athletes. This good ink would be fed to the journalists who worked for a daily newspaper (both broadsheet and tabloid), were freelance, or worked for press agencies. When an athlete was successful, the BPA's team would develop stories around the quotes they had collected. This three-man team divided the sports so that, at least in principle, there was 'coverage' of all events.

What the BPA had not considered was the idea that the audience for each publication was distinctive. In other words, the journalists did not need large amounts of information on events about people about which their readership had very little interest. What they needed was eye-catching material. Small stories that could make a point were required. The point, more often than not, was simply '*I was brought up to believe I could do anything*' (Balding 2004; Henderson 2004). Such sugary-sweet headlines for Paralympic sports were much in evidence during the Athens Games. Headlines such as '*Meet the Real Olympians*', which were fashionable during the Sydney Paralympics (Robinson 2000), were still dominant in Athens. '*Athletes in front line of campaign to change perception*' (Pryor 2004b) was a different take on the same theme. The majority of articles produced during Athens still had a 'feel good' factor associated with them, but headlines had a more explicit sport focus (Buckland 2004; Pryor 2004c). It remains to be seen whether reports from the Paralympics in Beijing 2008 will begin to mirror in style those written during the Olympics.

By investing in beat reports, the publications that had journalists at the Paralympic Games were giving legitimacy to both the IPC and the BPA, since both organisations produced the predictable copy that is the lifeblood of print journalism. It would appear that reporting on sport for the disabled is a double-edged sword. The athletes say that 'We want to be treated like anyone else' (Hind 2000), but this can be seen as journalistic handcuffs:

On one side, they will be dealing with athletes craving respect for their achievements, not merely acknowledgement of their courage and commitment. Yet, at the other extreme, the reporter who strays beyond the well-established territory of feel-good stories and heart-breaking profiles and dares to make a critical assessment risks automatic censure.

(Hind 2000)

Traditionally coverage of the Paralympics, both in the written and visual press, is laden with an appreciation for what the athletes have achieved before they get to the starting line. Most of the articles written by the journalists who acted as my informants during the Athens Games were edited to 'smooth the rough edges'. However, when an article went to press with a negative slant on the performance of British athletes, this antagonised the BPA's press officer. The report suggested some of the British long-distance runners were 'past their sell-by-date'. It was shocking to be confronted by a booming voicing asking:

Who the **** does he think he is? Those guys are so committed to their training and have done so much for Britain. [A journalist] has no right to write that sort of thing. If you say too much of that sort of thing he will lose the BPA's support!

What became clear was that this press officer felt that this negative article had undermined his work as a spin-doctor for the BPA. The press officer for the BPA was attempting (not unlike any other press officer) to control the dissemination of information about events as they unfolded at the Games. Most journalists who cover the Paralympics do not write negative material, and therefore it must have been a minor shock that went against everything he had worked for. What is interesting is that if a journalist on the beat for a major able-bodied professional sporting events questioned the quality of a star's performance when they 'let their side down', she or he would be seen to be doing their job. Those looking after the 'best interests' of the Paralympic Movement are more sensitive to such negative publicity.

Overall, press officers at the Paralympic Games worked diligently to provide positive facts to journalists in order to help shape stories. As Athens is two time zones ahead of the United Kingdom, journalists working for the British press could file stories well after the day's competitions were over, thus reducing stress levels. Working for a weekly meant that stories could be submitted as they were prepared, enabling editors to choose those that they thought were appropriate as far in advance as possible. The rest of the time was spent on the collection of the actual 'meat and potatoes' of journalism. Obtaining unique quotes was seen as paramount to good journalism. However, press conferences seemed to be the least likely place to get good copy.

Press conferences

The IPC ran a number of press conferences at the Games that, in effect, were live and interactive press releases. At one particular press conference, which was designed to be a celebration of the launch of the Paralympic World Cup to be held in Manchester in May 2005, questions were raised that challenged the validity of the event. One journalist questioned whether a World Cup could run as an invitational event that would exclude some of the world's best athletes. The answer given was that since the BPA was hosting the event (on behalf of the IPC), which included half a day's competition in cycling, swimming and athletics as well as four team tournaments in both men's and women's wheelchair basketball, it had to include British interest. In all the events, except women's wheelchair basketball, Britain had athletes worthy of competing. The Women's British wheelchair basketball team finished out of the medals in Athens, and as a result the mini-tournament was held without the presence of any of the Athens medal winning teams – thus making a mockery of the term World Cup. When numerous members of the press pointed this out, the curt response to these questions spoke volumes.

Press conferences are, of course, designed to do one of two things. The first is to act as a way of controlling damage to an organisation or an individual, as illustrated by the cases of high-profile sporting scandals involving the use of performance-enhancing drugs. There had been this sort of press conference in the past surrounding the Paralympic Games (Davies 2004), which often is hidden from view when the Games are represented in syrupy terms that belie a lack understanding of the culture of the Paralympic (sub)culture (Balding 2004; Howe 2004b; Howe and Jones 2006). When the European Paralympic Committee launched its anti-doping programme, 'Doping Disables', in 2001 (EPC

2001), it was in the wake of eleven positive drugs tests at the Sydney Paralympic Games, in an attempt to alleviate criticism of the number of athletes 'cheating'. This press conference, while undertaken to avoid criticism, can actually be interpreted as a positive step since it is an acknowledgement that the Paralympic Movement is in fast forward to commercialism, which appears to be the ultimate desire of the IPC (Jones and Howe 2005).

The other kind of press conference in Athens was designed to produce 'good ink' for whoever was holding them. In the case of the World Cup 'launch', the questions of several journalists soured the proceedings a little but the tone of the event picked up over a well-presented buffet lunch that also included several complimentary glasses of wine. Several hours after the press conference and the lunch, those of us still in the vicinity of the media centre were presented with a watch by one of the official Olympic sponsors. The ritual of the gift (Mauss 1990) suggested that the IPC was trying to buy good press coverage.

Forms of payment for good publicity are obviously not unique to the Paralympic Movement. This does, however, run counter to the issues of authenticity and trust that appeared at the heart of the habitus of the journalists in the Athens media centre. Most journalists were looking for stories that were sensational and true, but also that did not alienate institutional sources such as the IPC and the BPA. The desire to get a sensational story might be two-fold – to elevate the status of the journalist within his or her news organisation or, more altruistically, it might be a desire to see Paralympic sports get an increased level of exposure. In either case, it is important that journalists do not alienate their sources (Rowe 1999). One seasoned Paralympic beat journalist said that over the last decade he had established a detailed 'beat round' where he would always go and catch up with key informants (on a daily basis during the Games) to determine whether they had heard anything of interest. In this respect the role of the beat reporter is similar to an ethnographer – the longer you have been on the beat or in the field, the better and more effective your informants are likely to be.

The difference with the Paralympic beat is that because of the perceived sensitive nature of the topic (Hind 2000), journalists are not expecting to get a scoop. In fact, most of the stories that were filed (or rather the stories that made it to press) were either reports on results of events or small biographies. Connections with inside sources established through long service to the beat can be more reliable than those individuals who work within the press office. This is because the press office can be seen as a product of promotional culture (Wernick 1991), at the heart of which is a discourse that promotes and markets all aspects of contemporary society. Lines between entertainment and acts of promotion become blurred within this cultural milieu. The IPC has a desire for constant promotion that requires positive media coverage, including an agenda full of press releases and news conferences.

Getting good copy

Distinctive quotes taken from the 'horse's mouth' were highly sought after by the Paralympic journalists. General facts and information can be gathered from the BPA or IPC in the form of regular press releases, but a good quote that is distinctive to your story can inject life into an article and even improve its position within the paper. In Britain, the back page of a paper is more often than not the front page of a sports section (unless the paper has a separate section for sport), and a good quote often leads to a provocative headline which might mean that your copy makes the front of the sport section. In reality, of course, sport for the disabled often fills 'newsholes' in between coverage of male professional sports that vary across both national boundaries and the seasons. As the name suggests, these are literally small spaces in the paper where a short article may be appropriate, or sometimes even smaller gaps where a brief paragraph would suffice to draw attention of readers to an event.

Time spent as a rookie journalist working the Paralympic beat facilitated a culturally informed reporting, since I had lived experience of the Paralympic (sub)culture. *Run, Jump and Throw*, as a weekly publication, covered many of the same stories that other more seasoned journalists in the newsroom covered in some form or other in their daily papers. Therefore, it was important that the articles filed for *Run, Jump and Throw* had a degree of uniqueness and added authenticity. In the social environment around the newsdesk in the media centre, there was continual discussion and bartering as to what was likely to be today's story. Seasoned journalists who had worked the Paralympic beat before were always on the fringe of any discussion, while the novices, either in terms of the Paralympic beat or in terms of experience with journalism at major international sporting events, allied themselves with the BPA press officers. This was achieved through the physical proximity on the newsdesk, and by the fact that they were asking for advice and information each time a press release was made.

On the one hand there were the 'seasoned' campaigners, and on the other there were those who were new to Paralympic sport. In this dynamic between the BPA and the various types of journalists, the anthropologist working for a 'weekly' was very much a marginal figure in a liminal space (Turner 1967, 1969). The anthropologist was not in the same camp as the BPA or the seasoned or novice beat journalists but rather betwixt and between, thus facilitating an opportunity to learn the habitus of journalism through the hexis of being on beat.

For journalists who came to Athens from countries that do not have well-funded National Paralympic Committees such as the BPA, the IPC provided press releases on a very regular basis. These were statements of 'fact' that the world's journalists could use to shape stories they might want to develop. The journalists who relied upon the IPC for inside stories did, however, find that the information was often not focused on any one nation, so they would have to engage in more leg work in order to gather details for their 'audiences' back home. One of the key tools the IPC used at the Olympic Stadium was what they called flash quotes, which were quotes taken from medallists by a member of the IPC press office after their event had finished, in an area known as the mix zone. It was in this area that journalists were at liberty to interview the athletes after their competition. The IPC would often get quotes from athletes who were not being interviewed by other journalists.

A good journalist plays a waiting game in the mix zone in order to get a distinctive quote. Many of the British journalists were obviously after quotes from the same athletes, and would lunge at their victorious fellow citizen en masse. The press scrum which often ensued meant that many went away with the same quotes. By hanging back, the seasoned journalist was able to 'grab' a distinctive quote after the media scrum had subsided and just before both the athlete and the journalist went their separate ways under the stadium. It is worth noting that several journalists suggested that they never went to the mix zone but rather 'shaped' the quotations that came from the BPA or IPC press releases. The mix zone becomes an extension of the IPC's structural authority over the process of media output; by controlling the shape and size of the mix zone, the IPC limits contact with athletes that ultimately helps to shape stories.

In spite of the way in which the IPC and the BPA controlled the mediated outputs of the Games, I was still shocked upon my arrival home to find that even those journalists with experience of several Paralympiads were still recycling the old myths. As I wrote in my field notes on my return

Brighton, UK – Sunday 3, October 2004
Having just returned from the 12th Paralympic Games in Athens where I worked as a journalist for *Run, Throw and Jump* I struggled to focus on my Sunday paper. As my morning caffeine fix slowly worked through my bloodstream I could not believe what I saw before me. Clair Balding, known around Britain as a sporting commentator for the BBC, who has 'spread her wings' from being an expert in horse racing to all manner of sporting activities, had written an article for my Sunday paper. She had just been the anchor for the BBC's coverage of the Paralympics in Athens as she had four years earlier in Sydney. Writing in *The Observer*, Balding penned a patronising and paternalistic reflection of her experience that would not do Paralympic athletes any favours in the quest to be taken seriously. The piece, entitled *'The Games I'll Never Forget'*, appeared on October 3rd 2004, and it caused me such great offence that it marks the only time I have actually written to a media publication to complain. Balding writes as follows:

> It is impossible not to be affected by the Paralympic Games. Nothing crystallises more clearly the power of sport to change lives, to motivate, to bond people together, to bring out their inner strength. For all my intentions to think of it as any other sporting event, I have come away knowing more strongly than ever before that it is not. It has a purity of intent, a lack of commercialism, a feeling of 'family' to it that sets it apart.

The challenge now for the International Paralympic Committee, and their president Phil Craven, is to maintain that relative innocence while improving the standard of competition. Many want the Paralympics to be treated as if they were the same as the Olympics, but Craven is not one of them. 'This event is unique,' he tells me, 'and I want it to remain so. I'm all for elite competition and top-class sport, but I do not want to lose the crucial element of fun.'

This sense of 'fun' is not apparent if you engage in a critical ethnographic examination of the Games in Athens. If the actions of the current IPC administration are anything to go by, creating a 'fun family Games' thankfully is not on that organisation's agenda either.

In the build-up to the Games I was asked by the *Run, Throw and Jump*'s editor to write an article that highlighted two athletes from the Great Britain and Northern Ireland team as well as two international stars to draw readers' attention to the forthcoming Paralympics. One of the international stars I wanted to spotlight was my friend Earle Connor. Earle is a Canadian above-the-knee amputee who held four world records and was in 2003 awarded the World Disability Sports Person of the Year at the Laureus Sports Awards – sport's equivalent of Hollywood's Oscars. When I called Earle to ask for an interview, he put the phone down on me. Thinking there was a fault on the phone line I sent an email related to setting up an interview – which I assumed would be a formality – only for him never to reply – in time for my deadline. My piece on 'who to watch' at the Paralympics did not include Earle. In the excitement of attending the Games, I actually forgot about my friend and failed to send a follow-up email.

But when I got on the plane for Athens the reason for Earle's unwillingness to communicate became all too clear. Reading from a complimentary copy of the *Daily Telegraph*, I saw the headline 'Canadian fails drug test'. The article in brief reported that

> [t]he XII Paralympic Games suffered its first shock yesterday when Canadian Earle Connor, one of the most glamorous athletes here, was revealed to have tested positive for nandrolone and testosterone last month. Connor was immediately suspended from Canada's Paralympic team.
>
> The amputee athlete claimed he had been using a medically prescribed patch which helps normalise testosterone levels after one of his testes was removed because of concerns over cancer.
>
> Connor, 28, explained that he had been taking prescribed medications after being diagnosed with a severe gastro-intestinal infection at a competition in Germany in July.
>
> Connor, who holds four world records, has been suspended pending the final review of his test by the Canadian Centre for Ethics in Sport.
>
> Connor, who lost his left leg aged three months after a fibula problem,

won a gold and silver in the T42 category in Sydney four years ago. 'The Canadian Paralympic Committee is disappointed and saddened by this situation involving Earl Connor,' said Brian McPherson, the Canadian Paralympic Committee's director general. 'We hope that the matter will be concluded as quickly as possible so the focus can turn to the outstanding performances of the athletes on Team Canada.'

Connor had been one of three Canadian athletes nominated to carry their country's flag at last night's opening ceremony.

(Davies 2004)

It transpired that my friend had been caught up in a drugs scandal at the time when I was trying to contact him about the impending Paralympic Games. Though I was personally disappointed in his lack of virtue in regard to engaging in illicit doping practices, this 'high-profile' case marked a coming of age for the Paralympic Movement.

This coming of age illustrates why the 'fun and family' remark from Balding is so misplaced. As I wrote in reply to *The Observer*:

[Balding's] comments with regard to the 'family feeling' of the Paralympic Games are patronising in the extreme. To the athletes involved they are every bit as serious as the Olympics or any other high-performance sporting event. Yes, my family did attend the games to support my efforts (just as family members support Olympic athletes) but that is the extent of the 'family' experience at the Paralympic Games.

The suggestion that there is a sense of camaraderie that does not exist at other events suggests that Balding has little understanding of what it means to be a high-performance athlete, able or disabled.

(Howe 2004b)

The following was omitted from my published reply to Balding's article – no doubt due to word limit!

As for the Games being 'innocent' the seven positive drug tests at Athens on the back of eleven from Sydney four years ago indicate that the Paralympic Games have long lost their innocence, if indeed this was ever a feature of this event.

Paralympic sport is not innocent. The IPC's pursuit of a higher commercial profile and the desire of athletes to win increasingly valuable medals means that the Paralympic Movement no longer resembles the mediated image it is enthusiastically fostering.

For the Paralympic Movement lurks the danger of becoming top-heavy, of concentrating ever more energies and financial resources on fewer rather than on the equally deserving majority. The sensible chord of overall social responsibility and accountability should thus continue to be the guiding light of the Paralympic Movement. This does not always appear to be the case as concerns the ever-resource-hungry-elite-high-performance-sporting-system.

(Landry 1995: 14)

Summary

The IPC and its national affiliates, such as the BPA, controlled the newsroom information at the Athens Games. With press releases or conferences, both the IPC and the BPA were in a powerful position to control and shape stories through the use of these tools. These structures create a boundedness which is then subsequently articulated through reporting as a (sub)culture. The collection of quotes and, ultimately, the production of good copy are at the heart of the culture of sport journalism, but structural barriers imposed upon journalists at the Paralympic Games makes the goal hard to achieve. Much of what is written is a result of the rigid structure imposed upon the (sub)culture of Paralympic journalism that largely sees the distinctive cultural context of Paralympic sport as irrelevant. In these respects, the print journalists covering the Paralympic Games might be covering any other sporting spectacle except for the ultra-positive style that is adopted in the vast majority of stories that are published. The style of journalism has begun to shift away from the headlines that celebrate the triumph over adversity to a more sport-focused format. Headlines are changing, which is a step in the right direction, but arguably do not go far enough. Content in print journalism covering Paralympic sport should be as free to expose the distinctive culture that is a derivative of mainstream high-performance sport. A form of journalistic 'freedom' will ultimately lead to better reporting of the (sub)culture of Paralympic sport. Through the IPC, the Paralympic Games has become a high-performance spectacle worthy of good quality media coverage that necessitates the exposure of 'warts and all'.

Part 2

Impairment, sport and performance

6 The imperfect body and sport

The whistling you can hear is the back-rush of years to Victoriana. We still live with the Elephant Man school of thought it appears. Because people are different, because they do not consign to the norm, they must be kept behind closed doors. What arrant, distasteful, wicked nonsense.

(Mott 2000)

This sentiment is all too pervasive for many high-performance participants in sport for the disabled. The public discourse is about these attitudes being distasteful, but by and large in practice they are still rather self-evident in the manner in which disabled athletes are patronised by the fact that Paralympic athletes are not more involved in the organisational structures of Paralympic sport. While the last chapter highlighted an increased interest from the media in covering Paralympic sport, this chapter explores the relationship between bodily imperfection and the practice of sport.

High-performance sport in the mainstream 'able' world regularly articulates sporting accomplishment on a hierarchy where perfection is the aim. Commentators regularly refer to 'stellar performances' as being perfect or faultless, yet perfection is in fact unattainable. No one, as the old adage suggests, is perfect (Stone 1995). Until recently media coverage of the Paralympic Games has been limited, in part because of the unwillingness of the those who control the media to cover sport that is distinguished by its lack of perfection (Goggin and Newell 2000; Thomas and Smith 2003; Howe and Parker 2005). With its roots in rehabilitative medicine sport for the disabled (see Chapter 2), an activity initiated by an 'able' population draws attention to the physicality that is lacking in impaired populations who engage in sporting practice.

In this regard, DePauw (1997) examines how sport ostracises the impaired and argues that we need to re-examine the relationship between sport and the body as it relates to disability. Since the body demarcates the disabled as different, scholars within disability studies who have and continue to champion the social model of disability regard the body as material to the oppression of the disabled community (see Oliver 1996; Oliver and Barnes 1998). The fundamental importance of the body to the practice of sport may also be the reason that sport is an almost non-existent field of exploration within disability studies.

Since the early 1990s critiques of the social model have been more regularly expressed by scholars who have felt that the model needs to include more discussion of impairment, and therefore the body. In addition there is a perception that the Marxist values upon which it is based have little salience in society today (Shakespeare and Watson 1997). More contemporary ideas regarding disability suggest that a view of disability that is embodied more accurately reflects what is necessary to understanding the disabled community:

> It is possible to tread a path that challenges the disablism of the sociology of the body on the one hand, while utilising phenomenology to overcome the social models' disembodied view of disability on the other. We would argue that an embodied view of disability can provide a basis for a sociology of impairment.
>
> (Patterson and Hughes 1999: 599)

This chapter seeks to explore the importance of an approach to impairment that is embodied, and how it can be constructively used to explore the world of sporting 'imperfection'.

Theoretically, this can best be achieved by using the practice theory of Bourdieu (1977, 1990a) that conceptualises the distinction between the practice of social actors 'on the ground' and the large structures and superstructures that act to constrain the practice of actors but can ultimately be transformed by them at one and the same time. Bourdieu accomplished this by arguing, in different ways, for the *dialectical*, rather than *oppositional* relationship between the structural constraints of society and culture on the one hand and the 'practices' – the new term was important – of social actors on the other (Ortner 2006: 2). In particular, it is Bourdieu's embodied concept of habitus (Howe 2004a), where the lived body takes centre stage, that is of greatest importance when exploring the cultural practice of the Paralympic Movement generally and IPC athletics in particular.

The body of Paralympic athletes (and others involved in sport for the disabled) is constrained structurally not only by their culture but also specifically by the institution of the IPC, as well as the distinctive practice community (Howe and Jones 2006) of which it is a member. As well as structural influences of the IPC and other organisations, such as the explicit act of determining eligibility of bodies through the process of classification, the physical act of training the body for elite sporting performance must be seen as an embodied project. After all, 'embodiment is our life-long obsession. Eating, sleeping, washing, grooming, stimulating and entertaining our bodies dominate our lives' (Seymour 1998: 4). In order to fully appreciate the sporting practices such as those associated with the Paralympic Games, the concept of embodiment needs to be brought into the analysis. Kimayer has suggested that

The anthropological use of the metaphor of embodiment serves to maintain a place for the richness of bodily experience and significance of bodies as agents and areas of action. Embodiment works against the tendency to treat bodies simply as property (my body and yours) or as vehicles entirely subordinate to our will. The essential insight of embodiment is that the body has a life of its own and that social worlds become inscribed on, or sedimented in, body physiology, habitus, and experience.

(Kimayer 2003: 285)

From a methodological perspective, embodiment postulates that the body is not an object to be studied in relation to the cultural world but is the subject of culture or the existential ground of culture (Csordas 2002). This chapter adopts an embodied approach to explore the habitus that surrounds elite sport for the disabled, and is key to understanding how this sporting environment, through individual bodies, can be shaped and manipulated to serve the needs of the IPC. Importantly, the bodies of athletes with a disability may be seen at times as re-embodied. According to Seymour (1998: xv), '[r]e-embodiment takes place in a context of crisis, danger, fear uncertainty and risk. Although damaged bodies represent these characteristics in vivid form, they merely highlight the features that constitute the context of "high modernity".' In the context of this current research, I am using the term re-embodiment to illuminate what occurs to those individuals who are impaired through a trauma after birth. These individuals attempt to come to terms with their impaired bodies, and one vehicle they may adopt in the rehabilitation process is the practice of sport. For the congenitally impaired there is no explicit act of re-embodiment, as any change that may occur in their bodies is more gradual (e.g. the increase in strength through the process of weight training).

Habits of training

Adoption of habitus of high-performance training of the body is not indistinct from much of the work that has examined the body in the social world (Merleau-Ponty 1965; Bourdieu 1977, 1984, 1992; Leder 1990; Shilling 2003 [1993]). The exploration and analysis of habit illuminates the concept of agency as important to a practical and embodied praxis. In other words, the physical manifestation of culture through embodied action is fundamental to exploring the importance of the body in the context of sport. In the context of sport for the disabled for those who are involved in the practice due to a trauma, they have a second chance to rethink their bodies. Seymour suggests '[d]isability thus not only provokes reflection on the body, but also presents them with the opportunity to remake their bodies in different, and maybe less restrictive ways' (1998: 20).

Physical action that becomes embodied in certain situations may be seen as habitual, and these acts are often drilled into an athlete through countless repetition that lacks imagination. This can take the form of kicking drills in football, or sprinting drills in track and field athletics. Habitual acts that are further developed by improvisation can be considered dispositions (Howe 2004a). A disposition is an underlying tendency or propensity to act in a certain way, and therefore is more flexible than the habits that result from the learning of rudimentry drills. However, a disposition is still achieved without conscious thought before the action. The disposition is the embodied ability to put the habitual training together in such a way that it can be quickly adapted to suit any situation. Our disposition will suggest that we are likely to act in a certain way given a particular social situation. This distinction between habit and disposition is useful in that it explores the notion of human intervention in the sporting environment. When an athlete goes through the training regime required of an elite distance runner, his or her body habitually knows the 'race pace' simply by the 'feel' of the body; there is no need to rely upon a stopwatch. Changes that occur within a race, such as the tactics of the other competitors and the ability of the athlete to respond, are directly linked to the disposition or the ability to improvise that the athlete innately has developed through physical training and lived experiences more generally.

Merleau-Ponty's (1962) conceptualisation of corporeal schema is also of importance when trying to determine how athletes (and other actors) make the decisions they do without really thinking about them. When athletes make a strategic move in a race, they do not have to think about running or accelerating in a sense they 'know without knowing'. According to Crossley (2001: 123), 'The corporeal schema is an incorporated bodily know-how and practical sense; a perspectival grasp upon the world from the "point of view" of the body.' The embodied knowledge that the corporeal schema entails needs to be excavated in order to establish how Paralympians understand the cultural environment around them in times of training and competition.

The relationship between an agent and the environment cannot be explored independently of the idea that the environment at some level is subjective to the agent (Merleau-Ponty 1962). Therefore, perception of the environment and the relationship with the actor's body is then seen as an embodied activity. As a result, the members of the Paralympic Movement are being phenomenological because the act of interpreting their body is ultimately a reflexive practice. Borrowing from Nettleton and Watson (1998: 6), 'The reflexive self is one which relies on a vast array of advice and information provided in a myriad of sources'. As a result, the inspection of the habits of training for their specific sport allows elite disabled athletes to understand the world around the sport and to make sense of how their habits that are taken for granted may lead to them being sidelined from participating.

Every action of sporting performers embodies a structure and logic that is distinctive to their sport and the level at which they engage in it. As such, Merleau-Ponty (1962, 1965) and Bourdieu (1984, 1988, 1993) are useful allies. For Bourdieu, an athlete's habitus is the embodied sediment of every encounter he or she has had with the social world. It can be used in the present to mould perception, thought and action to the extent that it has an important role to play in decisions that an agent might make in future encounters. In this sense actors in general and, in the case of this research, elite disabled athletes specifically can be seen not simply to follow rules but also to bend them in much the same way as Merleau-Ponty (1962, 1965) conceptualises improvisation as being fundamental to an individual's disposition. Dispositions or, more generally, forms of social competence may be seen as a product of well-established social environments. In other words, while society may be seen as shaping agents, it needs individuals' improvisations from time to time if it is going to evolve. Therefore, in the post-industrial society in which we live it is as important to see the body as much a product of the self as it is of society. It is the self that provides improvisation by drawing upon the sediment of previous social encounters. In the case of the athletes involved in the summer Paralympic Games, the training regimes that they engage with as well as the 'fear' of being excluded from the next big international event as a result of changes in the competitive programme and/or the occurrence of injury (Howe 2004a, 2006b) means that the dispositions developed through being part of the Paralympic 'family' facilitate the ability to draw upon sediments of knowledge that ultimately enhance their membership within the Movement.

While the habit-forming nature of training is key to the embodied practice of sport on the international sporting stage, within sport for the disabled and Paralympic sport in particular the embodiment is less than able.

The 'less-than-able' body and sport

'Achievement in wheelchair sport does not have the power to transform the primary status, that of patient. Disabled sport remains sport for people with damaged bodies' (Seymour 1998: 115). As Seymour suggests, the bodies of impaired athletes have continually been judged in relation to some able-bodied 'norm', and the standards of play and performance are compared with those of mainstream competitions. This can have an adverse effect on participation rates within sport for the impaired, because sport is a cultural environment where a lack of physicality can lead to social inequality (DePauw 1997). Therefore, disability is an issue for the impaired individual on a number of levels. Importantly, an awareness of living in one's impaired body is a gendered experience. Men who have physical, sensory and intellectual impairments face a threat to their masculinity (Gerschick and Miller 1995). The complete and strong, aggressive, muscular body is the most tangible sign of maleness. Sporting bodies represent a pivotal form of 'physical capital' for disabled men, more so than for disabled women, because physicality has traditionally been considered an admired male trait. Of course, the issues relating to women's experiences of disability as it relates to sport are important (DePauw 1997; Hargreave 2000), but there is no room here for discussion of the impact of gender upon the body other than to say that disability, in my observation, leads to the feminising of the physical capital of even masculine bodies. In fact, countries such as the United Kingdom, Canada and Australia have produced the most celebrated

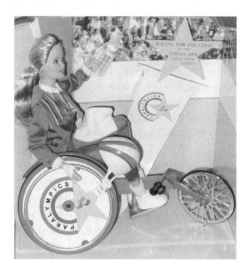

Figure 6.1 Barbie's friend Becky (photo by author).

Paralympians of recent times, all of whom have been women embodied – Tanni Grey Thompson, Chantel Petitclerc and Louise Sauvage (Howe and Parker 2005). The women who are Paralympic celebrities might be the reason for the launch in 1997 of a Mattel Inc. doll called Becky, who uses a wheelchair and who is designed to be a friend of Barbie (see Figure 6.1). When it was realised that the toy world was as inaccessible as the 'real' world, Mattel set about redesigning Barbie's 'Dream House' to make in accessible for Becky. The Sydney 2000 Paralympics re-launched Becky in a racing chair.

The body of Becky is the same as Barbie's, but she is in a racing chair – suggesting that the aesthetically pleasing look of the doll is still of importance. Development of this specialist doll highlights the concept of physical capital (Bourdieu 1984), and is a result of his awareness of the body's importance in structures of dominance and as the bearer of symbolic value. In spite of the feminine doll highlighted above, muscularity is felt to have high physical capital, and as a result men who are T54 wheelchair racers are perceived as the functional elite (Seymour 1998). For this reason, athletes with an impaired body become aware of their difference if for no other reason than by comparing physical performance with that of their 'able' peers. Because of the fear of the impaired falling behind 'normal' individuals, parents, teachers and coaches have unknowingly hindered the development, socially and physically, of young impaired individuals by creating what could be termed achievement syndrome or 'super crip' – the idea that the impaired are successful in spite of their disability (Berger 2004). It is alarming that scholars working within the study of sport for the disabled have unwillingly contributed to what I call 'super-cripisation' – the manifestation of the super-crip concept. In 1995 DePauw and Gavron published *Disability and Sport*, which at the time was the most comprehensive sociological text in the area of adaptive physical activity. This text was formatted to include 'cameos of achievement' that highlighted stars of sport for the disabled. Such a format might have had some validity at this point in the development of the sociological analysis of sport for the disabled, but to repeat it in the revived second edition is a retrograde step. Both DePauw and Gavron have an awareness that athletes with a disability want to be treated as sports people first and foremost (see DePauw 1997), yet by producing these cameos they ultimately contribute to the super-cripisation of Paralympic athletes – a process that characterises the ill-informed media outlets highlighted in Chapter 5. It is hoped that future social cultural work on sport for the disabled will avoid this pitfall.

My initial experience in an international event for athletes with cerebral palsy highlights the media's tendency to super-cripisation of Paralympic athletes. The limited attention the Canadian team received was couched in this way. This involvement forced[1] me into a disabled environment after a lifetime of being 'othered' but, lacking the social awareness of that fact, I was for the first time confronted by the realisation that society felt that I belonged with people with similar impairments. Initially when I was selected to represent my country at the World Games for Cerebral Palsy in Gits, Belgium, in 1986, my reaction was – 'great, I've never been to Belgium'. My field notes written at that time highlight a different frame of mind once the team had settled into the Games accommodation:

> Well here I am at my first World Games. I have worked so hard to get here but I feel ill with anxiety. Can this physical sign be my nerves over competing and doing my best for Canada or a direct result that after a week in the company of the rest of the team – I do not feel disabled – not like these guys anyway – I just don't seem to belong?

The whole experience surrounding my initial involvement was coloured by physical discomfort. My performances at this event were good, thus perhaps eliminating at least partially any associated upset due to performance anxiety. The discomfort may have in fact been due to the fact that my self-identity was questioned. My impairment made me for the first time part of a disabled group. I had in school been 'othered', but this situation was different. My body and its lack of normality mean that I was teased by fellow students, but I was socialised by my parents and teachers to see this as normal. In the environment of the Canadian Cerebral Palsy sports team, the whole group stood out as impaired – and as such my bodily imperfection became an issue in defining my belonging. These feelings are not unique to my experience, and may stem from a fear of being associated socially and physically with imperfection.

> I knew that instinctively that to be seen in the company of other disabled persons – especially people with an intellectual disability – meant being associated with failure, weakness and 'otherness'.
>
> (Camilleri 1999: 846)

In part these issues are related to the fact that only certain bodies are seen as successful. According to Seymour (1998: 119):

> A winning wheelchair athlete is seen as the epitome of rehabilitative success. The vision of the strong male bodies competing for honours on the sports field is an image that has currency in the able-bodied world. Bravery overcoming the catastrophe of a damaged body is a quality everyone can admire.

This image extends to amputee athletes who have also suffered traumatic injuries and use prosthetic limbs that can be used to enhance performance (see Chapter 7) and also provide the opportunity for re-embodiment that is not available to individuals who are congenitally impaired.

It is often rather difficult for the general public to see ability in some of the performances of individuals with impairments. As Seymour (1998: 124) suggests,

> While paralysed people may find inspiration in the sporting feats of other people with disabilities, the 'trickle-down' effect may be less than imagined and few able-bodied people would aspire to being in such a position.

The result of this can be stigmatisation of a young person who is interested in sport, and it may, perhaps more importantly, also have an effect on how sport for people with impairments is structured. The conundrum is clear – elite sport is concerned with enhanced bodily performance, yet how do you show this with a collective of impaired bodies?

The disabled athletes' physical performance at the Paralympic Games or any other major event will never be 'better' than that of able-bodied athletes. Although wheelchair racers do 'run' faster then the able runner, the physical act is not the same. We have to get away from the embodied notion of performance if our sport as a whole is to be taken seriously. Herein lies the problem – on the one hand a research agenda surrounding an embodied or an impaired notion of sport is important in accurately highlighting difficulties in how sport has been examined to date. On the other hand, if we compare impaired sport with 'able' sport in terms of enhanced bodily performance it will be undermined. One way around this conundrum is to redefine the concept of the elite sportsperson, where the concept of elite is based on training and not performance. I would suggest that the term 'elite' might better reflect the making of sacrifices in the training process, similar to an able-bodied serious amateur athlete. By constructing the concept in this manner, by shifting the focus away from performance to preparation, it may be seen as related to the social construct of the disciplined body as outlined in the work of Foucault (1977). As a sporting community, however, the impaired must operate within the hegemony of sport and challenge its values and concepts from within. Paralympians can challenge the prejudices that restrain the impaired in sport and the society it mirrors. This, however, can only be done if those in charge of the sport have this as part of their agenda (Howe and Jones 2006).

The bodies of impaired athletes are highly visible, in part because of their distinctiveness that might be perceived as abnormality. The embodiment of the abnormality can be seen in the movements surrounding a team's preparation for a major international event. The next four sections will look at the distinctive habitus and corporeal schema of athletes with a disability in the process of preparing for, travelling to and living at major competitions.

Badly adorned bodies

One of the initial entries into my diary regarded the arrival of my first national team uniform – a special occasion in every budding international athlete's career. It is worth quoting this moment during June 1986:

> It arrived in the post today, my uniform for the upcoming CP-ISRA World Games that are to be held in a month's time in Europe – Belgium to be exact. To my horror, when I tried the uniform on nothing fitted properly. Everyone who has ever ordered anything from a mail-order clothing company no doubt has had a similar experience. Why can clothing manu- facturers not standardise sizes? A men's medium singlet/running vest should be the same size from whichever company you order it, regardless of where it is made in the world. This uniform is special to me in part because of the significance of the World Games. It symbolises all the hard training I have put in with the view of being selected to run over the middle distances. In the end, my mother skilfully and lovingly altered the uniform, so that it ended up fitting quite well. By the time I wore it full-time (during the train- ing camp – prior to departure in mid-July) I was really proud to be repre- senting Canada.

The symbolism tied to the adorning of the athletes in uniforms at international sporting festivals is of course not an advent of sport for the disabled. Identifica- tion with symbols, such as uniforms, to some marks the pinnacle of achieve- ment, but to others it represents negative elements associated with nationalism. The Canadian Paralympic teams have never had the same uniform as the Cana- dian Olympic teams. While the joint sponsor of the Canadian Olympic and Paralympic teams, Roots, produced both uniforms (2000, 2004), the quality and quantity of the Paralympic uniform was inferior. While publicity called the Par- alympic uniform 'distinctive', the fact that it was not the same as the Olympic team's was considered problematic by many athletes. As one athlete suggested, 'Yes, the logo should be different for the Paralympic team, but the uniform should have the same number of pieces and be the same colour and design.' This lack is disappointing for most Paralympic athletes, because the same team uniform represents equality – the idea that a Paralympic athlete's performance matters as much as that of an Olympic athlete. When the uniform is worn, it is the literal embodiment of how the nation understand its athletes. Issues of nationalism not withstanding, the acquisition of one's first national team uniform is an important moment – hence my initial disappointment when it was received in such an ill-fitted form. However, I was not alone.

On arrival at the training camp I found that most of the other members of the team had suffered the same fate regarding their uniform size selection, but many of them had been unable to get theirs altered. A collection of Canada's 'best' athletes with cerebral palsy were staying at a camp on the University of Windsor campus, and by and large we looked as a group as though we had been dressed in the cast-offs from a charity shop that specialised in red and white clothing. This visible spectacle was not enhanced by the nature of the impairment of cerebral palsy, which entails part of the body being affected by varying degrees of spasticity. This manifests itself in shaky walking or frequent stumbling for ambulant members of the team. The team also had members in wheelchairs, where lower limb spasticity was less obvious but it was still present in the upper extremities. Ill-fitting team uniforms only highlighted the embodied difference of the team, shaping its habitus and the treatment we received from those outside this group.

This awkward embodiment not only has an impact upon the aesthetics of an individual or team of athletes who are impaired, it also influences the manner in which an athlete may train. My experience of training has always been the same as that for an 'able' runner, although my performances could not be as fast as for athletes that did not have an impairment who trained to the same intensity. The biggest difference occurred when my body began to fatigue. I would lose my balance, often tripping and falling. These accidents were never graceful, and the 'road rash' on the right side of my body was 'refreshed' every couple of months. Scabbed knuckles on my right hand – the result of my body's right side going into a spastic state – were more embarrassing than painful, but were a hardship I had to bear in order to run fast. Depending on the level of their involvement, other athletes with a given impairment might have their training altered more substantially. For example, athletes in wheelchairs who throw the shot or discus do so without moving their lower limbs – they are secured in the throwing circle in their chair to given them a stable base from which to throw. Today the technology has developed so that wheelchair athletes use a throwing frame (see Chapter 7) which allows them to develop more force.

On the whole, an elite performer competing in sport for the disabled should train as hard as an Olympian, with certain variations to allow for the individual impairment. This does not mean that training should be any less strenuous. However, this is not what I observed in 1986:

> After several days on the campus at Windsor, completing our final training preparation, I began to realise that many of the track and field coaches that were travelling with the team knew little about high-performance sport. The workouts they were setting for the athletes seemed inappropriate for the events in which they were competing, particularly in relation to where

these athletes should have been in their competitive schedules. Coaches seemed to want all the athletes on the national team for specific events to engage in the same form of training during the camp, regardless of how that fitted in with the schedule developed by the athlete's individual coach. Some of the athletes were treated as pets because they were personally coached by the national coaches, and as such the training at the camp was more appropriate from the point of view fitting into their schedules than it was for athletes who were outsiders, such as myself. The most striking observation about the training of the athletes was how unfit they were generally, as well as specifically for track and field athletics. This state of affairs may be a direct result of the fact that many of them also competed to an international level in other sports such as swimming and football (soccer).

Specialisation in a particular sporting practice was not considered a necessity by those who organised the national teams within sport for the disabled in the 1980s, both in Canada and other leading nations. In a very real sense this was an amateur movement – sport was about participation, not performance, and the efficiency of the bodies of many athletes was not ideal. The practice of serious leisure (see Howe 2004a), where a sportsperson pursues his or her interest with the vim and vigour of a professional, while not being paid for the pleasure, was the approach adopted by no more than a quarter of the athletes involved in my first World Games. In part the training of these athletes was because they were participants, and as such they were treated as pets (Bale 2004) and not like well-bred race horses. The team generally embodied recreational athletes who were more interested in the social elements of international competition that they were in achieving in the sports arena.

Because I took my sport very seriously the lack of focus by many of the other nation team members made me feel an outsider. This was exacerbated by the travel to events. The movement of a large number of people for an international event requires establishing a degree of control over individual bodies. Establishing a team habitus is difficult since membership is fluid but there are certain elements of travel to events became habituated.

Travel to events

To those looking in from the outside, one of the highlights for an elite athlete with a disability most certainly would be the travelling far and wide in search of improved performance and medals. However, exploring the world because you have a talent can easily be romanticised. Travel to distant shores as a tourist, however, is not the same as being transported to another sporting venue in some far away location for a race or competition. In fact, for some athletes going on another trip can be seen as a hardship. The travel between one's home and competition venues can at times be rather disruptive to an athlete's life and to their physical well-being. Not only may athletes be leaving loved ones behind for, at times, months on end, but there are also physiological factors related to flying that can impede high-quality athletic performances. Even if athletes are away from their homes and training bases for a short time, the effect of what is commonly referred to as jet-lag can hamper performance. Jet lag occurs when you travel across numerous time zones and your body often feels unusual for at least a day per time zone travelled. In reality it takes a finely tuned athlete less time to accommodate to their new surroundings, but it may still impact on their performance.

The travel itself was nothing out of the ordinary, although for anyone who dislikes flying the necessity to travel as a team means that extra stress is involved in such occasions. The fact that a large number of people wish to check-in at an airport on mass is not that unusual – if you go to major airports around the world, you can often see large tour parties congregated in cramped environments waiting to be called to the gate for the flight. In the case of a Paralympic team, however, there is the added frustration of the paternalistic attitude of society regarding individuals with a disability. The paternalism that follows individuals with a disability is embodied by limiting freedom and responsibility by well-meant regulations which, in the context of travelling as a team, means that team officials look after all the tickets and passports and the group is strongly encouraged to travel together. There may be valid reasons for the groups travelling together, such as deals with the Paralympic Games official carriers etc., and these are no doubt why Olympic athletes often travel together (at least on a squad basis), but in the case of the Canadian Paralympic Committee the attitude to many of the athletes was to treat them like children. Many of the athletes suspend their social role when travelling with a team and, though not ill, adopt a Parsonian 'sick role' (Parsons 1951). The concept of the sick role, in the simplest terms, means that a person's normal social role, whether that be a mother, father, student or elite athlete, becomes temporarily suspended when he or she is ill. While none of the athletes travelling with the team is actually ill, nonetheless their normal social role is temporarily suspended while administrators from within the travelling contingent care for their basic needs. Adoption of the sick role was key to a stress-free trip in the early days of my involvement with sport for the disabled. It was a vital part of the athletes' habitus.

The majority of athletes that have been Paralympians from the 2000 Sydney Games onwards are very unaccustomed to adopting the sick role. Yet there are factions within the disability sport movement that still to this day have an ethos that is grounded in paternalistic principles and the sick role. Travelling to the Robin Hood Games, which in 1991 were the unofficial CP-ISRA World Games, I was acutely aware that I felt a bit like a sheep, a member of a flock mindlessly following people through the airport. In my mid-twenties and having just finished a Masters degree, the feeling of being led around the airport terminal in Toronto was foreign. I felt like an outsider liminal to this social world, and yet my field notes identified that there may have been good reason for this type of travel arrangement:

I am beginning to get very frustrated with being shepherded about the airport terminal but to my surprise many of the athletes seem content. We were due to arrive at the airport four hours before the flight was due to depart. The airport is a madhouse and those in charge of the team seem to have little clue what is going on – talk about 'hurry up and wait'. The act of getting a large group of people ready to travel anywhere can be really drawn out but other travellers are giving us a wide berth and staring, often with looks of disgust. Most of the athletes have adopted the 'sick role' and with bodies that are to a varying degree – imperfect – not simply a result of the impairment (cerebral palsy) and its resulting spasticity but also due to the fact that it is hard to believe over half the team are athletes. As a collective, we do not look like Canada's finest athletes. We look like an institutional group setting out on holiday.

There is a real resentment among a handful of the athletes that we are being treated as children who need to be looked after on this 'big adventure'. What is clear is that there are many athletes on the team who have seldom been away from home. Many of these individuals are older than myself, but they appear 'helpless' and the comings and goings of the terminal building are all at once both frightening and amazing, yet this physical environment was quite natural to a small group of us. We had our passports and tickets taken away – for fear that we might lose them. It might make sense if it helped speed up the check-in process – in the manner that it is done with some holiday package tours – but we still had to wait in line to have our luggage weighed.

This treatment resulted in a team-management approach that can best be characterised by the phrase articulated above – 'hurry up and wait'. It was important when engaged in team travel to adopt the habitus associated with the sick role and therefore reduce the stress. The anger at the 'hurry up and wait' approach to travel was counterproductive. Anywhere the squad travelled during my time as a member it was a long drawn-out process, and there were certain segments of the group who looked completely frustrated. From my earliest involvement, however, there was a large constituent of the group who were bewildered in a fashion that was akin to Dorothy in *The Wizard of Oz*. Team-management strategy implied that it was easier to treat all the athletes as being child-like because, in airports and other transportation outlets, there seemed to be fewer surprises of luggage left behind or unattended if each athlete was treated the same. Most people have experienced the anxiety of putting luggage through check-in at an airport and wondering whether it will end up on the same plane as you. These concerns are amplified if you are travelling in a large group of disabled athletes to a major championship.

Packing bodies

The athletes' luggage at times has to be treated with kid gloves. It would be disastrous if a squad of athletes were to show up without their competition equipment. For high-performance athletes, equipment that is used in competition is of vital importance. Able-bodied athletes also need to worry about technical equipment such as various throwing implements and items like pole-vault poles that need to be stored in the cargo hold of the plane. Competitive footwear such as throwing shoes or track spikes can easily be placed in hand luggage. However, if luggage does not arrive safely, new implements can be relatively easily obtained. The equipment used by athletes with a disabilities is more technically specific (see Chapter 7), in part because it is an extension of the body – particularly the legs – in the case of wheelchair and prosthetic users. Over the past twenty years these chairs have become very sport-specific, and as such have helped with improved performance. Importantly, these chairs are built to fit a specific athlete, limiting as much as possible his or her impairment. Such personalised development takes months to get just right, and as a result the loss of a racing chair before an event is disastrous.

Athletes who use a wheelchair to compete cannot simply load their racing or playing chairs (in the case of tennis, rugby or basketball) on the plane in the hand luggage. Each chair comes in a large travel crate, which means by and large that the chairs are stored with the rest of the onboard luggage. Because the wheelchair athletes cannot have this vital piece of equipment with them on the plane they suffer a greater degree of stress than most passengers because of the personalised nature of a competition chair. Will it arrive on time? Will it still be in one piece? The situation can be even worse when, because of the size of some of the wheelchair crates, they need to be shipped a day or two before the athletes. Not only does this mean that athletes will be more uncertain as to whether or not the luggage will show up at the team's destination; it also means that they are forced to take a break in their training for up to a couple of days. Most of the top competitors may have several competition wheelchairs, each one designed to fit like a glove. Chairs are often replaced when there is an advance in technology, perhaps when the next generation of racing or playing wheelchair is made of a new material or there might be a new theory about improving the aerodynamics. The time and money involved in getting the chair just right means that an athlete gets very attached to his or her equipment, and leaving it, albeit well packed, in the hands of airport staff must certainly be difficult.

The same degree of anxiety can be felt by athletes who compete in leg-amputee classes. It is probably worth noting that many leg-amputee athletes choose to contest events from wheelchairs on the track (class T54) but, for those who do not, placing racing legs in the cargo hold also must take a leap of faith. Today each leg is specifically designed to help the athlete be as biomechanically efficient as possible. Individual fit around the position of amputation is tried and tested to produce the best performance possible.

Each Paralympic athlete is aware of the risk associated with carried performance tools in the cargo hold of a plane. Young athletes learn from old to how best protect their legs or chairs. Secure packing to avoid the risk of damage is also part of the habitus of travel for athletes with a disability. With a bit of luck, all the required baggage will arrive with the team. Once the team arrives at its destination, there is more waiting around the airport than might normally be expected. It is not just the usual traffic through customs or the collection of luggage; teams are also required to obtain the accreditation that is needed in order to gain access to the Games village. Paralympic Games accreditation is similar in many ways to a military 'dog-tag', in that it replaces conventional identification such as passports and other travel documents whilst athletes, team and competition officials are resident in the village. Everyone that is a member of the Paralympic 'family' wears this identification (normally around their neck), in a similar vein to those who are involved with the Olympics. The Para-lympic 'family' is a catch-all term used to describe athletes, competition offi-cials, classifiers, and members of the executive of the IOSDs and the IPC, as well as the paid employees of the latter, but (as Chapter 5 highlights) it has nothing to do with a familial environment during the Paralympic Games (Howe 2004b).

Travel as a team to the Paralympic Games may be seen as the embodiment of (dys)ability. Here I use the prefix *dys*, from the Greek meaning bad or ill, as it has been effectively used in social theory of the to refer to the *dys*-appearance of bodies when they are in pain (Leder 1990; Howe 2004a). The process of travel-ling as a member of a team creates a habitus, but this will not be entirely dis-tinctive to elite sport for the disabled. Adoption of a sick role is perhaps easier for impaired athletes when they are healthy, since many of them have been through a rehabilitative programme at one time or other (see Chapter 2). Sitting around being herded from one place to the next illuminates the social component of impairment that is (dys)ability. In other words, while athletes with impairment are not seen individually as patients, as a collective they are the embodiment of such.

Arrival of 'patients'

Even before the era of heightened international security following the events of 9/11 in 2001, getting accreditation could be a long and drawn-out process – especially after a long day of transcontinental travel. After travelling from Toronto to Los Angeles and then to Seoul, South Korea, for the 1988 Para-lympic Games, the Canadian contingent was exhausted. The team had stopped overnight in Los Angeles, where members of the whole team congregated before taking the thirteen-hour journey across the Pacific Ocean to South Korea. By the time the team arrived in the small hours of the morning, the airport was largely deserted. This made movement through customs rather easier than had been expected, since there had been a degree of social unrest during the Olympic Games a month earlier. The Chief de mission[2] had warned the team in advance that the process could be heavily delayed. Much of the team was processed through the accreditation system quite rapidly; however, a number of us were delayed by four or more hours because either there was no record of us taking part in the Paralympic Games or the information the officials had implied that we were not the people we said we were – for example, the person I was to be rooming with in the village, who was an ambulant cyclist, was meant to be a wheelchair user according to officials in Seoul. This discrepancy in classification meant that this particular athlete had to go through the rigours of reclassification before he could get his accreditation that would give him access to the Paralympic village. In this particular case the athlete was given a temporary accreditation, until he was officially classified that afternoon in the village.

When the team has begun to clear accreditation, the process of loading athletes on to buses begins. Thankfully, once the team has claimed their luggage this is loaded on to trucks to be delivered to the Canadian section of the village. With so many wheelchair users in any multi-disability sporting environment, it is imperative that those in charge of ground transport provide buses that are accessible. While event organisers are aware of the importance of this today and major games have suitable transport, back in the mid-1980s there was a clear indication that the Parsonian 'sick role' might be more closely linked with competitors in sport for the disabled that were present to participate than would be considered appropriate today. On the arrival in Belgium of the CP-ISRA World Games, the transport to the 'village', which ended up being a residential institute for the physically disabled, was a series of ambulances:

> The travel to Brussels was not too bad. Since the plane was only half full the team was able to spread out. In spite of seeming to wait forever in the airport before departure, everything went smoothly. It was rather alarming that initially that we got on the plane forty-five minutes before the other passengers. We seemed to be marked out for 'special' treatment, and when we arrived in Brussels we were loaded on to a series of large ambulances. I can understand that they might not have many wheelchair-accessible buses, but there seems to be a symbolism associated with this form of transport. It is almost as if a disability means that a person is ill; that the purpose of their existence is to be a patient.

It is clear that symbols such as ambulances transporting athletes with a disability make members of that community question social attitudes. On one level, the practicality of this type of transport for a large number of athletes with impairments is important for Games organisers. There is also a stigma associated with travelling in an ambulance, and therefore those who do so might be perceived as the embodiment of patients.

In the first instance, it is important that transportation be flexible enough to accommodate numerous members of the team who are in wheelchairs. These vehicles in Belgium had a limited number of fixed seats, and three-quarters of their space was dedicated to positions where wheelchair users could be strapped in safely after being loaded on to the vehicle using the mechanical lift. On many occasions ambulant athletes have been forced to stand for hours on end during the journey from the airport to the Games village. The factor that distinguishes the use of local ambulances (at Games more recently, regular buses have been used with several rows of seats removed) is that it sends out a message to the public that there is something wrong with those who are travelling in this type of vehicle. An ambulance is a vehicle that is used by paramedics to take people to and from hospital, and as such it suggests there is something wrong with those who need them. In Belgium these ambulances were more akin to the vehicles used by disability charitable groups, which suggests that those inside are in need of support, care and attention. While this is not a message many of the athletes of today would feel comfortable being associated with, some rather enjoyed this new form of attention – fitting happily into the sick role, a transformation within the athletes on the team that took me by surprise. Once the team had been picked up and transported to the place where they were staying, the athletes became more dependent on the support staff as well as the coaches.

Paralympic village life

Anyone who has been to either boarding school or university, or indeed lived in an 'ordinary' family, will be well aware of the compromises that are required to live communally. Living in the communal environment of a Paralympic village is distinctive from all of the above for three reasons. First, the assemblage of teams at the Paralympics means that the village is always completely international, and as a result life in the village is multicultural. The second reason the village is a distinctive environment is that the group of people are congregated together because of a competition. The other reason is that while these villages are not traditional institutional environments, attempts are made to make the buildings accessible environments. As highlighted in Chapter 2, the village in Seoul in 1988 was less than ideal with regard to access to buildings, etc., but it was a vast improvement on the residential environment used during my first World Games in 1986:

> The team was housed in this residential school/hospital in rural Belgium south of the city of Brugge, where Flemish is the native tongue. This was an isolating environment. Although the rural location made it ideal for training it became claustrophobic, since this site was away from the competition venues, so our only company was our fellow team members and our competitors. Sleeping in a classroom on military cots with eleven other guys was also an unrestful experience. Some of the athletes had picked up colds, which meant they were coughing and hacking all night. Others had smuggled alcohol from home and would go out after the curfew and get violently ill, and still others would sneak off for a romantic rendezvous with someone on our team or someone whom they had just met – no doubt improving international relations. With all of this going on it suggests that the members of the team were by and large 'normal', but it was frustrating to those individuals who were there with the express purpose of winning a gold medal. It was all a bit of distraction. In a

positive sense, though, it was no more distracting than it was for our competitors. On top of this, the food was distinctive – traditional Flemish – which took sometime getting used to, but it did provide those who were looking for them with yet another excuse for a bad performance when the competition began.

This transition in the inability of my early team-mates to manage their own affairs might have been a direct result of the fact that many on the team had never travelled aboard before (or no further than the continental United States, which has many cultural similarities to Canada). The team had pitched up at a residential school-cum-hospital that at the time was reminiscent of a Dickensian institution where there was a curfew and poor food, and we were staying twelve to a room. The support staff (other than the coaches) that were charged with caring for those individuals who were more severely impaired were often notable by their absence, leaving fellow athletes in the role of carer. It became clear that there were a lot of hangers-on in the official team party. For these Games, where each athlete had to raise the finance to attend (a local Rotary service club was a tremendous help to me in this regard in the early days), some of the support staff had their expenses raised by the athletes they were there to support. Everyone was in the same predicament at major games, and if you were going to be successful in the competition then it was necessary to block out the confusion of village life. Although for most living in the village is simply a matter of being housed close to the venues for the games, for athletes who are there to perform the stresses of village life can either enhance or destroy expectations. On many occasions the 'sick role' placed upon my body had a negative impact on my performances, in part brought on by my desire to record the distinctive cultural environment that was opening up before me.

The reaction I had to the imposition of the 'sick role' being placed upon me is not dissimilar to the feelings expressed by Murphy (1987) in his classic monograph *The Body Silent*, where he chronicles his re-embodied life with paralysis:

> [Paralysis] can be congenital or it can happen at any age, to people of widely different social circumstances. The similarity of our condition is, however, social, for no matter who we are or how we got into our unenviable situation, the able-bodied treat the physically handicapped in much the same way. Disability is defined by society and given meaning by culture; it is a social malady.
>
> (Murphy 1987: 4)

The bodies of sport performers with a disability need to be trained, clothed, transported and housed in order to compete internationally, but how does this impact upon the less than able body?

Summary

Bodily 'imperfection' makes the Paralympic athlete communitas distinct. There may have been a misguided attempt, by those in the media, to empower this sporting community by using discourse related to performance and achievement, which is non-embodied. By incorporating discussion of the distinctive habitus of disabled sporting culture into media coverage the public's 'education' might be accelerated, increasing their understanding of difference and encouraging further their financial support.

The Paralympic Movement is gradually helping to change society's perceptions. The battle for recognition of elite performance by severely disabled athletes has to be waged. If the sporting movement as a whole gives into the IPC's vision of a streamlined minimally disabled Games, the sport will essentially be no different than its able equivalent. Control by the communitas of former and current athletes over the transformation of the Paralympic Movement is required, since

> The transformation of sport culture will mean when we are able to 'see' sport and athlete with a disability without seeing any contradiction, without assuming a physical liability, stigma or deformity, and without assuming an impaired athletic performance. That is, we will see an athlete, an athletic performance, and a sporting body.
>
> (DePauw 1997: 428)

While current social theory has over the last decade been largely influenced by work on the body and notions of embodiment, if equity is ever to be achieved for the impaired in the sporting arena, research has to be refocused. Whether this means altering the current paradigm associated with sport or transforming it completely is unclear. However, as long as the body is the focus of sport, we will continue to be seen as less than able. 'A person with a disability may perform "incredibly well for a person with a disabled person", but a damaged body can never achieve the physical capabilities of a body that is undamaged' (Seymour 1998: 124).

7 Technology and the Paralympic Games

Earlier chapters have established that classification within high-performance sport for the disabled has an important cultural political influence on the Paralympic Movement. Classification of bodies determines whether someone is eligible for Paralympic competition. Those who are eligible can benefit from technology that enables the remaking of their impaired bodies. The impact of technology is felt particularly strongly in the new commercial environment that is key if the IPC is going to continue its 'progress' to be just like the IOC. Commercial influences are being exerted on the Paralympic Movement in the area of mobility technologies, since many athletes require the use of either a wheelchair or a prosthesis for general mobility and competition.

A discussion of the technological improvements in wheelchairs and prosthetic limbs will be used to shed light on how this technology is being employed to improve performances of elite disabled athletes and in turn reshape the cultural politics of the Paralympics. It is important, however, to remember that these technologies have to be purchased and therefore the Paralympic Movement represents a developing market. This chapter can best be expressed in the phrase 'techno-centric ideology' (Charles 1995). The desire of the athletes to perform with greater proficiency encourages those developing new technologies continually to seek improvements for the sporting practice. In other words, technology is literally pushing the Paralympic Movement forward. Finally the question will be asked as to whether the advances in technology are actually of benefit to the cause of empowering disabled athletes, and the disabled communitas at large:

> Technology and kinesiology are symbiotically linked. They have a mutually beneficial relationship. As technology advances, so does the quality of scientific research and information accessible in the field. As kinesiology progresses and gains academic acceptance and credibility, technology assumes a more central role in our field. The more scientific the subdiscipline, the more we can see technology at play.
>
> (Charles 1995: 379)

Following this statement, it is clear that the field of high-performance sport has benefited from an increase in technologies that have been developed to harness the power of the human body (Davis and Cooper 1999). This is perhaps most self evident in the Paralympic Movement by developments in technologies associated with mobility, namely the wheelchair and prosthetic legs. Able-bodied high-performance athletes rely on technology in their day-to-day training (Hoberman 1992; Shogan 1999), yet when these athletes perform in sports like athletics the technology that has got them to the sporting arena may be completely absent from view. Able-bodied athletes do take technology with them to the start of an Olympic final, as their clothing and footwear are products of advanced technology. However, specialist clothing and shoes appear less like advanced technology in comparison with racing wheelchairs and space-age prosthetic limbs, as they are not explicitly aids for mobility. In the case of the wheelchair 1500 m demonstration held at the Olympics, the technology for movement (the wheelchair) is explicit:

> When persons with disabilities use technologies to adjust the participation in 'normal' physical activity, the use of these technologies constructs this person as unnatural in contrast to a natural, nondisabled participant, even though both nondisabled participants and those with disabilities utilize technologies to participate.
>
> (Shogan 1998: 272)

Technology such as racing wheelchairs and flex-feet (artificial legs biomechanically designed for running) have enhanced the performances of athletes whose impairments benefit from their use. It is these two technologies that I will briefly explore in this chapter before discussing the technology used by athletes with a disability who need assistance of a more explicit technical nature. Importantly, these technological aids, whether used by the impaired public or by Paralympic athletes, have an impact upon embodied experience, as highlighted by the notion of 'packed bodies' in the previous chapter.

The wheelchair

It has been argued that man has used various forms of technology to transport the sick and impaired since about 4000BC, and there is clear documentary evidence suggesting that medics in ancient Greece were prescribing various forms of transportation for the ill (Kamenetz 1969). The 'vehicles' were not designed to be self-propelled, and the first known ancestor to what we would recognise as a wheelchair did not appear in Europe until the seventeenth century, when it was used as much as transport for the wealthy as for the ill:

> [I]t is evident that wheelchairs have a long association with medicine, up until the early 20th century *wheeled chairs* often intersected the divide between a mode of transport for the wealthy and a medical apparatus for injured, sick and/or disabled people.
>
> (Woods and Watson 2004: 407)

The focus of rehabilitative medicine in the early twentieth century was to rid individuals of impairment. Continued use of a wheelchair denoted an explicit sign of failure (Woods and Watson 2004). The use of a wheelchair either signalled the failure of rehabilitative medicine or, more worryingly, the user was believed to have given up of the process of returning to 'a normal life'. The stigma of using a wheelchair is evident in the fact that it is only in the past fifteen years that most Western nations have made it a legal requirement not to discriminate against individuals with physical impairments. Importantly, the symbol to denote that a building, a car-parking space and public transportation are accessible is a graphic representation of a person in a wheelchair.

The patients at Stoke Mandeville hospital in the 1940s who became the guinea pigs for the use of sport as a method of rehabilitation were all confined to wheelchairs (see Chapter 2), and as such all the early events in the development of sport for the disabled were organised and regulated for users of this particular mobility aid. Early sporting wheelchairs were less mobile than today's standard-issue hospital chair, and it was not until the 1990s that international standards were put in place for the way in which a 'day' wheelchair should be constructed. However, athletes with a disability began to build sport-specific wheelchairs during the mid-1970s. 'No longer a multipurpose wheelchair for all activities, the new wheelchairs target the performance requirements of specific activity and maximise the functional capacity of the athlete who has a disability' (Yilla 2004: 33).

In the mid-1980s, racing chairs were four-wheeled and cumbersome by the standards of today's 'space age' technology but were a great improvement on the technologies of the Guttmann era of the Paralympic Movement (see Figure 7.1). As already mentioned, this era celebrated participation over high performance, and it was not uncommon therefore for athletes to use the same chair for daily activity and for sporting competition. Specially designed sporting racing chairs may be seen as the first major step toward a high-performance Paralympic Games. Performances at the Paralympic Games had been improving with the turning of every Paralympiad, as a close examination of the athletics results from the IPC website will attest. The desire of athletes to move better and faster and also to assist in the production of technology by offering expert advice allowed them to achieve these aims, and no doubt accelerated the transition from a sporting pastime to an environment of high-performance sport. However, developing improved technology is only half the battle. First of all, technologies develop at different rates, and thus some nations might make advances in performance simply because of their access to superior technology. Medal tables at the Paralympic Games have been traditionally dominated by Western nations, in part because they are at the forefront of the technological revolution. Like the Cold War arms race, the Paralympic Movement quite literally, in the race to produce the most efficient and advanced mobility aids, has a 'leg race' on its hands.

On another level the development of new technologies allows athletes to train more efficiently with less risk of injury (Howe 2004a, 2006b). Moves to

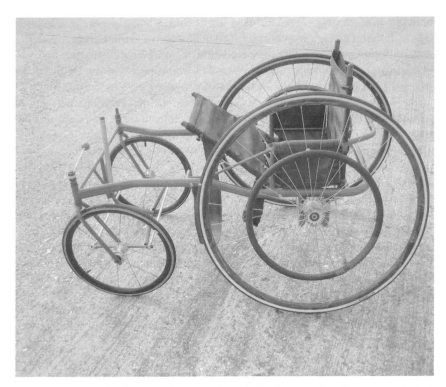

Figure 7.1 A Handcrafted Metal racing chair (*c.*1986), reproduced courtesy of Draft Wheelchairs.

transform the technology used for movement in the sport of athletics, the racing (wheel)chair and the static platforms like those used in throwing events can be seen as an attempt to use technologies to enhance the impaired body's performance.

Within athletics throwing events (discus, javelin, shot put and club[1]), wheelchairs have, since the early 1990s, been replaced by throwing frames which do not have wheels. These frames are more robust than a wheelchair, and as a result are easier to tie down to a solid position. The frame is tied to a series of points on the ground in a shot put or discus circle, or behind the line on the javelin 'run-up'. Each frame is specifically designed for the athlete, and as such enables him or her to get the most out of the throwing technique. Because of the complex nature of the technique associated with throwing implements such as the shot, discus and javelin, rules regarding seated throws have come under close scrutiny in recent years (Frossard *et al.* 2006). Some classes of athletes are not allowed to let their gluteus muscles to leave the seat of the throwing frame. Breaking of this rule has been increasingly been monitored by officials at top-level events, including the Paralympic Games and IPC World

Championships. Those throwers who are able to use their legs as well as their upper body ultimately face the prospect of being reclassified into a more able class, since the use of legs can be an obvious advantage in a sport where the longest distance thrown in six attempts establishes the winner. There has also been concern about the use of materials in the frames that allow for a 'spring-like response' to the throwing action. Athletes hold onto a pole that is part of his or her frame, recoil the body and then release the implement. Excess energy generated by this action cannot force the body outside the throwing area. In other words, if the force from the pole is so great it allows the body to break the plane of the throwing arena, the resulting effort will be considered a foul. What is important with regard to discussions about technology is that there is a strong correlation between 'the interaction between the design of the athletes' throwing frame and their throwing technique' (Frossard *et al.* 2006: 1). There is a direct link, therefore, between the impaired body and technology, to the extent that the technology becomes an extension of the body (see Haraway 1991).

With the increasing use of biomechanical analysis of throwing position as well as the use of more technologically advanced materials, athletes from all classes are producing better performances (O'Riordan and Frossard 2006). As previously highlighted, sometimes throwing events are held across classes using decathlon-type tables, which means that the winner may not be the athlete who throws the furthest but rather the one who scores the most points on the table for his or her particular class (see Chapter 4). This can be a particular headache for the event officials. While the use of tables means that there are fewer events on the programme of any major meet, the relative abilities of the athletes in multiple classes makes it more difficult to police whether athletes are properly classified or not. Some athletes might have a desire to take advantage of this complex situation and bend the rules, but this needs further exploration.

Perhaps the best example of the role of technology is the development of wheelchair track racing. Today's high-performance racing chair has three wheels (one less than those I first encountered in the mid-1980s), and is aerodynamically built of lightweight carbon fibre so that developing more speed takes considerably less effort than it did on the heavier models of two decades ago (see Figure 7.2). The frame is a 'T' shape, which provides stability through the long front and a degree of rigidity (Yilla 2000), both of which are required when the chairs travel at high speeds For events over 800 m, both men and women T54 are faster than their able counterparts. This is in part due to the fact that drafting is allowed in the IPC athletics rules. As a result, elite races on the track are similar (at least in terms of tactics) to road cycling, where drafting is an advantageous way to save energy. Racing machines with very thin, highly-pressurised tyres and a carbon-fibre frame that, year-on-year, weigh less and less, also benefit from a steering mechanism called a compensator. This is a technology that has been developed to allow wheelchair racers to 'forget' about turning their chairs through a corner. The compensator can be set to the direct the chair around the bend once it has been activated by the athlete. Compensators are fixed to the axial front wheel so that the athlete hits it upon entering and

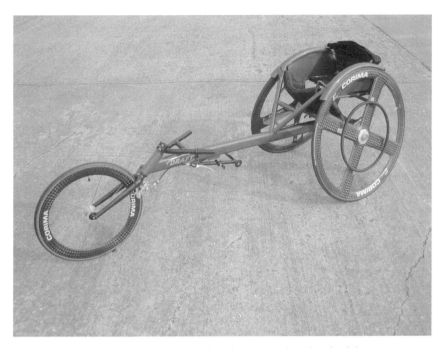

Figure 7.2 Racing chair from 2005, reproduced courtesy of Draft Wheelchairs.

exiting a turn. This is all the athletes have to concern themselves with (that is, apart from the art of racing) while on the bend. This technological advance has allowed racers to improve their performances markedly. Not only are their chairs lighter and more aerodynamic than ever, but they are also easier to handle.

Technology transfer

Remarkably, at the Paralympic Games in 1988 a large number of Canadian chair racers brought their old chairs with them to give to athletes from less technologically advanced countries. These chairs were well used, but were an improvement on some of the technologies used by countries who had just begun to be involved in sport for the disabled. This sort of recycling of technologies no doubt was not a unique Canadian concept, and I am sure other nations engaged in the practice as well, but Seoul was the first and only time I saw this happen. It may well have been a regular occurrence at Paralympic Games prior to 1988, but I cannot find any records that confirm or deny this fact. What is clear is that it is not a practice that occurs today – at least in such a public forum. There are two reasons for this. First, today's wheelchairs are built around athletes. In the past, a standard racing wheelchair was purchased and athletes added their own padding supports and straps so that they could create their own optimal racing position. Some chair racers like to sit on their legs, while other prefer their legs in a more conventional seating position. The position an athlete adopts in his or her racing chair is about getting the positioning appropriate to drive as much force as possible through the push rims.[2] Seating positions may vary depending on the type and severity of impairment. Today, chairs are custom built and there is no longer any need for extra padding or excess strapping. For the top racers, their chairs are now an extension of their bodies. As a result, the most successful wheelchair athletes can be seen as cyborgs – that is, 'a coupling between organism and machine' (Haraway 1991: 150). These athletes and all individuals who are accustomed to using a wheelchair for mobility, to the degree that moving in a wheelchair becomes habitual, develop a hybrid body (Haraway 1991: 178).

Transferring wheelchair technology means that the new user will need time to develop a understanding that is akin to a cyborg. In other words, athletes take time to get used to each wheelchair they own: 'Interestingly, the wheel-chair has assumed status and significance similar to the polo player's horse or the hockey player's ice skates' (Botvin-Madorsky 1986: 737). The other reason there may not be a wholesale transfer of used wheelchair technology is that the Paralympic Movement has moved on (some would say progressed) from its foundation in rehabilitative medicine that led to a model of sport that was primarily concerned with participation, to the high-performance model that takes centre stage today. Athletes and NPC are largely concerned with improving performances and winning medals, and as a result levelling the playing field by giving other nations yesterday's technology is not on the top of the agenda. Access to state of the art technology is the saving grace for many Western nations involved in the Paralympic Games. On the one hand, NPCs from Canada, United Kingdom, Australia and the United States might attribute their success to the better treatment of the people with disabilities in their countries. However, it is technology and not government policy that is keeping these nations at the forefront of the Paralympic Movement.

Government policies in relation to the disabled communitas, including the provision for sport, have been established not with the aim of enabling a better life but rather of appeasing groups that are marginal within society. Investment in Paralympic programmes should also not be seen as a hallmark of an enlight-ened society. Following Gruneau (1991: 177), 'hegemony works best when it concedes to opposition on the margins in order to retain the core principles upon which particular forms of dominance are sustained'. In other words, because most individuals with impairments (including athletes) are at the margins of society they are not in control of enough resources to fund pro-grammes as large as those of an NPC. Referring to those who control sporting practice, Morgan (1994b: 313) states:

> For as long as [the able-bodied] are able to marshal effectively the superior resources they command, it is almost always in their best interests to appear more compliant to the demands of 'marginalized others' than they really

are. That is why it is more accurate to characterize the negotiating posture of dominant groups toward 'marginalized others' as a calculative, manipulative one rather than a grudging conciliatory one.

While government policies are designed to keep the dominant group in a position of power, the act of Canadian wheelchair racers passing along last year's technology in Seoul in the short term has had a positive outcome. A T54 athlete who was recipient of a 'nearly new' chair only just made it out of his heat in the 100m in his own chair. After adapting the new chair he was a contender in the final the following day, finishing a close fourth. Was the act of the Canadian team selfless or selfish? By providing nations who were less developed in terms of sport for the disabled with technology for athletes to improve their performances, the Canadians can either be interpreted as giving these nations a helping hand or as leading them to become dependent on technology and therefore maintaining their dominant position. What is clear is that Seoul 1988 marked an important shift in the desire of the Paralympic Movement to be in pursuit of achievement sport (Bale 2004), as the technology of wheelchairs began to incorporate the improvements of minimal weight etc. that could be adopted from sports such as cycling.

Prosthetic limbs

Perhaps the most popular imagery associated with prosthetic limbs is that associated with the haggard old 'sea dog' who hobbles around on a wooden peg-leg. These wooden prostheses have a long history (Webling and Fahrer 1986; Chaloner *et al.* 2001), and are more than adequate mobility aids. The term *prosthesis* is Greek for an addition designed to remove physical stigma:

> Prosthetic medicine is dedicated to physical normalisation and is devoted to the artificial alteration of both function and appearance, but it enters the realm of biopolitics because it uses the 'normal' body as its tribunal and blueprint for action, and treats the impaired body as a spoilt entity that must be hidden and corrected.
>
> (Hughes 2000: 561)

In the context of sports participation as well as day-to-day mobility, one of the problems associated with traditional technology is the development of pressure ulcers and painful stumps that develop where the prosthesis joins the body (DesGroseilliers *et al.* 1978). Such dermatologic ailments are at their most painful during the process of rehabilitation, when part of gaining an ability to use a prosthetic limb means the skin at the point of contact needs to 'toughened up' (Rossi 1974). This is particularly acute for leg amputees, as the act of bearing weight on a prosthesis can create a good deal of pressure on the 'stump' that is the result of the amputation. Regardless of technological advances, the pull of gravity means that this pressure will always have to be dealt with.

The connection between a prosthesis and the upper body obviously does have gravity to deal with, but the lack of 'weight bearing' means that pressure ulcers and the like are less troublesome. Observations suggest that technological advancement associated with arm prostheses have not had an impact upon sport, since few leading arm amputees use prosthetic limb(s). This is not to say that there have not been improvements in arm prosthesis technology; rather that the arm is less important when it comes to performance enhancement. Yes, the loss of a forearm or complete arm can have an impact on running performance, and some athletes use a prosthesis to improve biomechanical efficiency – which is, of course, an element in performing well – but these prostheses are seldom more than additions to the body. In other words, there is little technological development that has gone into their use. For the non-athlete, advancement in technologies to allow the movement of prosthetic hands and fingers has greatly improved the quality of life for many amputees, but as yet this technology has not been seen as important to the enhancement of sporting performance simply because the vast majority compete with no prostheses at all.

Since 1988 there has been a marked improvement in the technology associated with leg prosthetics. The material from which prostheses are made has changed markedly from wood to fibreglass to all manners of carbon fibre and lightweight metals used in advanced scientific design. These mobility aids have been a product of state-of-the-art 'space age' technologies, and as a result the athletes who are the vanguards of this new technology are producing performances that would have been considered impossible twenty years ago. Technology has advanced with three aims in mind: to produce better performances; to increase the comfort for an individual, athlete or otherwise; and to enable an improvement in efficiency of movement. Advancement is most evident on the track, but also in field events where athletes with amputations have the option of competing as standing athletes or as athletes who use throwing frames, as highlighted earlier in this chapter.

For athletes with leg amputations it has been particularly evident to me over the last two decades how their stump has been cared for in the process of changing from walking legs to competing legs:

> I have been amazed to observe close at hand the ritualised preparation and treatment of an amputee's 'stump'. This is the generic name that seems to be used by most of the athletes who are amputees that have crossed my path. Many of the athletes have pet names for the point of amputation that range from friendly and familial to the vulgar; the nature of the name used no doubt is linked directly to each individual's disposition and how that varies depending upon the social and cultural context from which they come. Within the context of this, at the IPC Athletics World Championships [in Berlin 1994], where there are few women present, the lexicon associated with having a prosthesis is far from politically correct. What was interesting was how the point of impairment became such a focus of attention for this group. For athletes with a dis-

ability who have complete bodies, like myself with CP or the visually impaired or the spinal cord injured, there is not the same sense of connection with the impairment.

The reason amputees and in particular those who have lost all or part of their lower limbs turn the point of impairment into an object of discourse is that there is a necessity to have a paternalistic 'relationship' with this part of the body. Development of pressure ulcers, verruca of the stump, general chafing and blisters require that the stump receives constant care and attention. To the athlete for whom high performance is the objective, the 'stump' needs to be treated as a child that requires pampering.

Most of the complaints that a person with an amputation suffers from are the result of sweat and the resulting chafing (DesGroseilliers *et al.* 1978). The physical culture of running, let alone at the intensity required to be a Paralympian, means that the battle to keep the stump healthy and free from ulceration is an ongoing battle for elite athletes with this impairment. It is paramount that the stump is dry, for example, each time the prosthesis is worn. This requires constant monitoring by the athlete. Generous amounts of talcum power are used to keep the stump dry – so much so that one athlete suggested 'I should be sponsored by them. The talc keeps me blister free. I go through it like crazy and the number of athletes I suggest use [the product] it would be great if we could get some sort of kick back!'

Once the athlete coats their stump with talc or other drying agent, then a cotton sheath is placed around it before the prosthesis is attached. This is done with a combination of Velcro straps and buckles, depending on what best suits the athletes. Depending on the event, the potential for chafing is high. The more vigorous the workout, the more there is a need to look after the stump. For those athletes who have been involved in Paralympic sport for many years, their stumps become more resistant to all forms of ulceration.

Since the field notes above were taken, the care and treatment of stumps has improved tremendously. Cotton stump socks supplemented with a small gel pad that was used to cushion the end of the stump provided the next advance in technology. This innovation allowed athletes to achieve a more secure fit between the stump and the prosthetic limb. A gel pad soon became a gel sheath or sock that completely surrounded the stump. One of the problems with this technique was that although the gel sheath created an environment where the stump was protected, it could also be very warm and created a 'sweat trap' that could lead to many of the conditions highlighted above. Today many of the top of the range 'flex foot' legs are built around the individual's stump, and are secured in place by a vacuum seal device which often includes gel padding.

The use of flex-foot technology, that is the carbon-fibre blades that are used instead of the old-fashioned prosthesis (where flexion of the ankle was either mechanical or non-existent), is almost universal at the highest level of Paralympic sport. As a result there is little advantage to having this technology once you are at the Paralympic Games, but it is required to get there. Countries who are at the developmental stages of sport for the disabled programmes may find it unrealistic to train runners and throwers in leg-amputee classes, as the cost of up-to-date technology can be prohibitive. This is a clear downside to the race for more efficient prostheses which, with the proper training, can produce improved performances. Such technology is available only to those who have the economic capital.

On the other hand, for those who have access to the technology, and in a global sporting economy that is increasing, the culture associated with the use of prosthetic limbs has been transformed. When I first observed athletes with leg amputations in large numbers, they would wear a leg that was cosmetically similar to their unaffected one – the prosthesis was painted in matching skin tone with a sculpted calf muscle that was the mirror image of the other. Athletes did not go as far as having hair painted on their prosthesis if their leg in the flesh was 'decorated' in that manner, but considerable energy had gone into hiding the impairment. Today, as least within the culture of Paralympians, most athletes do not bother to hide their amputation behind a cosmetic limb. In fact, most elite athletes are happy to wear either a technologically advanced leg – which for the very best athletes will be supplied as part of their sponsorship deal – or a more traditional prosthesis that is adorned with graphic art often promoting either a brand of prosthesis or sporting equipment, and in some cases a national emblem. This art work makes the prosthesis highly visible when the weather is warm – as is usually the case during the summer Games – and could be seen as the result of these athletes being more confident of the validity of their sporting achievements and about their bodies more generally.

The performance standards have improved dramatically across the board within the classification of leg amputees, in a large part due to the increased accessibility, in the West at least, to state-of-the-art technology. At the Sydney 2000 Paralympic Games, Canadian Earle Connor, an above-the-knee amputee (class T42), grabbed many headlines by destroying the competition, many of whom at the time did not use the same technology as him. It has been said, however, that Connor was so far in front of his competitors they would need more than technology to be on level terms with him. Ironically, on the eve of the Athens Games in 2004 Connor tested positive for nandrolone and testosterone (see Chapter 5). It gives a certain salience to a comment he made in my company and that of other athletes during Sydney 2000: 'You are naive if you think that there are not athletes here doing drugs.' As a result of his drugs ban, Connor – who denies the use of drugs to enhance his performance – was unable to shine in Athens. Another star shone in his absence. A young South African, a double below-the-knee amputee, made the Paralympic world as well as the mainstream world of athletics take notice. Ultimately his presence made the athletics fraternity question when and if impairment becomes an advantage.

The 'Oscar Pistorius Rule'

Since the Athens Paralympic Games, one of the big stars of the Paralympic Movement has been a class T43 athlete named Oscar Pistorius, from South Africa. Oscar came to the Paralympic communitas's attention when he won the gold medal in the 200 m in world-record time in Athens, in spite of being a bilateral below-the-knee athlete. It was phenomenal to see him compete favourably with athletes who had just one prosthetic limb. Being a bilateral amputee, Pistorius has always competed in both T43 (both legs amputated below the knee) and T44 events (one leg amputated below the knee). There are usually not enough competitors in the T43 class, and as such he is permitted to compete in events for the T44. This class is more impaired than the class to which Pistorius rightfully belongs. His 100 m, 200 m and 400 m T43 world records are all faster than the T44 world records. Pistorius and his sponsors recognise that his achievement is in part down to the technology of his sponsors. Össur, the prosthetic manufacturer, states on its website:

> Oscar recognizes that Össur's Cheetah® running legs have helped him run at his fastest and accomplish this huge feat that has never before been done. The high energy return the Cheetah® blades offer help spring Oscar to his next step and past the finish line.[3]

Pistorius has been called 'The Fastest Thing On No Legs' (Philips 2005), and he has been seen by some as a breath of fresh air in the Movement for his refusal to see himself as disabled but rather as someone who does not have any legs. What is apparent to anyone who sees him run, however, is the level of balance he achieves in his running action, which cannot be achieved by athletes who have only one prosthetic limb. As an onlooker at the IPC Athletics World Championships which took place in Assen, the Netherlands, in the summer of 2006 stated:

> Oscar being included in a T44 event provides him with a clear advantage. You do not have to have a great knowledge of kinesiology to realise that an athlete who is symmetrical in their running style will be advantaged over an athlete who is not. Clearly a good T43 will almost always beat a good T44 on the track. The advantage is so clear to see. Just look at the motion of his 'feet' after he finishes running!

The blades that replace his lower legs and feet produce so much energy that when he runs down the track even after the race has finished the excess energy still causes bouncing. This does not happen with mechanical ankles.

Oscar has become a celebrity in the few years since Athens, grabbing headlines at the IPC VISA World Cup, which has been held three time (2005–2007) in Manchester, England. This is an event that attracts some of the world's top Paralympic athletes, and it was one of the first events on the

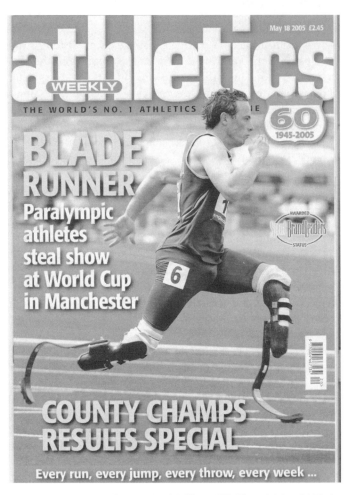

Figure 7.3 Oscar Pistorius on the cover of *Athletics Weekly*, 18 May 2005 (reproduced
with permission).

Paralympic calendar to pay travel expenses to 'star' athletes. Such was his
performance at the inaugural event in May 2005 that he graced the cover of
Athletics Weekly on 18 May with a headline 'Blade Runner' (see Figure 7.3).
Five days before these outstanding performances Pistorius had appeared on the
BBC's cult sports quiz show, *A Question of Sport*.

On one level it seems appropriate to celebrate the achievements of Pistorius – he certainly can run fast – but on the other hand his fellow competitors
may be disadvantaged because of the symmetry with which he is able to run.
Has the technology that produces his fine performances been an aid to his
performance? Balding provocatively suggests that Pistorius has been caught in
a speed trap:

Does he have an advantage over runners with normal legs because the spring in his carbon-fibre limbs gives him more elevation? Or is that cancelled out by the fact that he has no ankle flexion and no feet to propel him off the starting block? Put simply, is it fair contest, or does he have an unnatural advantage?

(Balding 2005)

Pistorius himself commented on the situation several years ago, stating that 'The IAAF started questioning whether a disabled athlete can run able-bodied times and now that has changed to whether disabled athletes should compete' (Balding 2005). The question remains whether his impairment offers an unfair advantage compared with 'able' athletes.

Certainly Pistorius cannot run without artificial legs, but discussion of the possibility of him competing in the Olympic Games in Beijing (Burnett 2005) has resulted recently in the IAAF taking action against what they call 'technical aids'. The press release related to the rule addition in the spring of 2007 read as follows:

IAAF Council introduces rule regarding 'technical aids' Mombasa, Kenya – 26 March 2007[4]

This afternoon IAAF Council concluded its study of all the Rule Change proposals which will be presented to the 46th edition of the IAAF Congress which takes place in Osaka, Japan on 23–24 August, just prior to the 11th IAAF World Championships in Athletics.

Although 143 proposals to amend IAAF Competition Rules were studied, Council decided to implement one new provision with immediate effect in accordance with its Constitutional powers under Article 6.11c and subject to confirmation by the Congress in Osaka.

The specific rule introduced in Mombasa, which will be numbered Rule 144.2, relates to the use of 'technical aids' during competition.

This new rule prohibits:

(e) Use of any technical device that incorporates springs, wheels or any other element that provides the user with an advantage over another athlete not using such a device.

(f) Use of any appliance that has the effect of increasing the dimension of a piece of equipment beyond the permitted maximum in the Rules or that provides the user with an advantage which he would not have obtained using the equipment specified in the Rules.

A Paralympian who is a 400 m runner commented recently:

[This is an] interesting new rule passed by the IAAF. I wonder if they'll call this the 'Oscar Pistorius Rule' in the years to come. He just ran 46.3 to come 2nd in the 400 m at able-bodied South Africa nationals and 46.0, a week earlier. The Beijing standard is 45.5 and he is starting to challenge that target. I can't imagine what else this rule would be addressing. It would be interesting to know how it originated.

What is clear is that there is a desire to keep the sporting body at least visibly pure. Technical aids such as 'flex feet' with their carbon-fibre blades do respond differently to the forces being put through them than does the more mechanical human ankle. Is it the intent of technology like flex foot to enhance perform-ance beyond that of the able-bodied runner, or is it simply designed to give the prosthetic wearer the most comfortable mobility aid? If the goal of companies producing technologies for impaired athletes is to improve on the 'natural' human body, then the IAAF may be justified in the implementation of this new rule. However, if Pistorius's achievements are simply the result of his abilities as an athlete then it appears there is clear discrimination taking place. Similar sorts of issues have been highlighted by Miah (2004: 166) when he states 'the way in which disability is separated from able-bodied sport may serve as some guide for how genetically enhanced (or deficient) athletes might be treated'. It could be argued, judging from the response of the IAAF to Pistorius, that Para-lympic athletes who use so-called technical aids may in fact be treated as 'cheats' within the mainstream sporting context. The fear is of course that '[o]ur bodies may be devalued and treated as machines, to the extreme where some technophiles may seek out a cyborg-like existence and declare the body obso-lete' (Charles 1995: 383).

Other bodies

The bodies that have been absent from the discussion of technology in this chapter are those that benefit from advances in sport science support – bio-mechanical and physiological, for example – but do not require a mobility aid such as the use of a wheelchair or prosthesis. Visually impaired, ambulant cere-bral palsy, and intellectually impaired athletes are able to compete in sport without the use of special technologies of mobility. The relative normality with which they compete can be seen to be detrimental to how these groups may be treated both inside and outside the Paralympic communitas. Athletes with visual impairment are relatively easily understood by the public. Every day, a high percentage of the world population wears visual aids. Many use either spectacles or contact lenses, which are designed to help people better to appre-ciate the world around them because to a degree a large portion of the world population is visually impaired. As our eyesight deteriorates as a result of spend-ing too much time at the computer or through the passage of time and old age, we can understand poor sight. As a result, athletes with visual impairment are not marginalised to the same extent as are those who have cerebral palsy or an intellectual impairment.

Regarding those whose impairment is more difficult to understand, such as the uncontrollable spasticity of an individual with cerebral palsy, or those whose physical manifestation of their condition is only evident in social environments – such as an athlete with an intellectual impairment – technological intervention will not manage their body so that it is restrained in a manner that is acceptable to the normality assumed of sporting practices. Following Shogan (1999), I would argue that the mobility technology used in sport for the disabled is unnatural in the context of high-performance sport, but in light of the 'super human' results achieved through the use of either state-of-the-art wheelchairs or prosthetic limbs, it has become an accepted currency over the last decade. In other words, in the media attention surrounding certain role models, the vast majority of whom are athletes with either spinal cord injuries or limb amputations, technical aids have become synonymous with Paralympic sport.

The use of technological aids has led to a litany of supercrip stories. According to Berger (2004: 798),

> '[s]upercrips' are those individuals whose inspirational stories of courage and dedication, and hard work prove that it can be done, that one can defy the odds and accomplish the impossible. The concern is that these stories of success will foster unrealistic expectations about what people with disabilities can achieve, what they *should* be able to achieve if only they tried hard enough. Society does not need to change. It is the myth of the self-made man.

In the narrative of these stories as they relate to Paralympic sport, there is often a lack of understanding of the habitus of Paralympic sporting practice. They also follow closely athletes who benefit from technological aids, as it is 'easier' to see ability in a fast one-legged racer or a wheelchair racer that can 'run' a mile faster than the current able-bodied world record. However, many Paralympians who are highly trained and motivated athletes but do not require these technologies can never live up to these ideals.

Summary

While the development of mobility technology that enhances sport performance is beneficial for the impairment groups concerned, it marginalises further those athletes that do not use technologies directly in their competitive performance. Because the high-end wheelchair athlete is able to perform at the same level or better than an able athlete, to the public the ability of these athletes is obvious. On the other hand, in an athlete that has cerebral palsy which affects both legs and who runs 100 m much slower than his or her able counterpart, it might be difficult to see their ability.

The possibility of new bodies for the disabled are provided by sport-specific technology. In elite sport for the disabled, there are increasing numbers of athletes with mechanical, artificially designed bodies creating new sporting potential. Technology has the capacity to 'normalise' the disabled body, to produce 'sporting cyborgs'. Those who have the most sophisticated aids are traditionally from the West, and they are the athletes who have the greatest chance of winning medals and breaking records. As a result, the Paralympics risk becoming a show of radical technology rather than a show of athleticism, leaving behind those from the developing world without performance-enhancing technology at their disposal. However, China was the leading nation at the 2004 Athens Games in terms of medals won. It is also reported that there are 60 million people in China with an impairment.[5] Rumours in Athens suggested that there were 50000 athletes competing in regional events seeking selection for the Athens Games. There were only a handful of wheelchair athletes on the track from China at Athens, but an established European wheelchair coach at the time stated that it takes four to five years to produce a world-class racer. In 2006 at the IPC World Athletics Championships, a high number of elite Chinese racers appeared suggesting that the China will be unbeatable in terms of medals won when they host the Games in Beijing during 2008.

8   Accommodating Paralympic bodies

> The developments at Stoke Mandeville have been credited with starting the international sports movement for disabled people. Rather than being idealistic about the values of disabled sport, we should remember that its modern organized roots were driven by political expediency. These do not lie in sporting values for themselves, but in the use of sport, competitive activities and rehabilitation practices as a method of transforming paralysed ex-servicemen into taxpayers.
>
> (Anderson 2003: 474–475)

The political expediency that Anderson highlights above is not only a feature of the past but also a currency that those with power within the Paralympic Movement spend in order to achieve progress today. But what is progress in terms of the Paralympic Movement? Is it the increased commercial support that is a by-product of 'improved' media attention? If this is progress to the IPC, then to a large extent the organisation can see itself as successful. Alternatively, progress could be seen as the fulfilment of the IPC's dictum *Empower, Inspire and Achieve*. This suggests the Paralympic Movement is concerned with empowering its athletes in the hope that their performances will inspire others to great achievements. The difficulty with this is that few athletes are empowered by a practice that was established for them. Perhaps more importantly, the relationship between the practice of high-performance sport and embodied imperfection is an uneasy one. Following Smith (1999), the reader needs to understand the power struggle that is ongoing between the athletes and the institutions of Paralympic sport – primarily the IPC. In this struggle, hegemony acts as

> a linchpin providing some sense of leverage between the historical role of power in giving form to human subjectivity on the one hand and the will and initiative of men and women on the other. It appears to politicise the more sanitised notion of 'culture' by planting the asp of power within its breast. It allows us to 'explain' the particularity of forms of conduct – cultural specificity, cultural difference – while retaining a faith in the dignity

of the (subaltern) subject: formed by yesterday's power, constrained by today's.

(Smith 1999: 233)

Sport is an embodied practice and a hegemonic battle field for those with imperfect bodies. As such, many people who possess less than normal bodies may shy away from the masculine physicality (Murphy 1987; DePauw 1997) associated with sporting practice. It is argued, therefore, that sport and athletic prowess are constructed in such a way as to alienate those, especially the disabled, who can neither aspire to nor achieve such standards. The complete and strong, aggressive, muscular body is the most tangible sign of maleness (Seymour 1998). Sporting bodies represent a pivotal form of physical capital, because physicality has traditionally been considered an admired trait. To those who have read this monograph from the beginning, it should be obvious that the primary form of otherness is the social construction of disability and its related embodied form impairment. This is not to suggest that issues related to gender, race or sexuality are any less important when examining the structure of sport, but simply that these issues require their own empirical investigation. Muscularity has high physical capital. Placing physicality as the key component of identity, this monograph has thus far attempted to establish a link between the degree of impairment and the liminal position (Turner 1967) of individuals within the Paralympic communitas.

Having a 'good' physique has a currency or value within wider society. Someone with an impairment who uses a wheelchair, for example, may not have the ability to develop a physique that is highly sought after in society at large. Not every 'able' individual can do this either, but such individuals possess a body that is 'normal'. For this reason the athlete with an impaired body becomes aware of his or her difference, if for no other reason than by comparing physical performance with that of their 'able' peers. However, as an impaired sporting culture develops, new image ideals of the body are beginning to become apparent. The chiselled torso of champion T54 wheelchair racers is a fine example of this. On the one hand this is a positive step – it shows acceptance of the impaired form. On the other hand, more severely impaired individuals might continue to be marginalised because they cannot meet this ideal. As Seymour (1998: 120) suggests,

> The preferencing of physicality in spinal injuries rehabilitation may disenfranchise the very people who most need its services. The creation of sporting heroes as rehabilitative triumphs obliterates from view the many severely damaged people for whom such activities will always be an impossibility.

By their very nature, sports celebrate physical skill and prowess. Impairments, however, are often exacerbated in an environment such as the competitive arena. Work in the field of disability studies has suggested that individuals with impairment are pushed to the margins of society (Oliver 1996; Thomas 1999), and therefore as a result of their involvement in sport could be seen as liminal to the practice. Media coverage of sport for the disabled perpetuates the liminality of the athletes by measuring their sporting endeavours in light of their disability. Their ability to overcome disability, rather than their athletic ability, becomes the focus of praise and admiration (see Chapter 5). Achievement cameos lead to a super-cripisation of Paralympic sport which ultimately clouds an accurate representation of the culture of the Paralympics by acting as a catalyst for the many errant images that are portrayed by the media. Headlines that broadly celebrate 'triumph over disaster' when the featured athlete is simply living with an impairment take away the celebration of pure sporting achievement that is the hallmark of mainstream sporting practice.

Hahn (1984) suggests that because sport for the disabled is based on physical tasks, those in this communitas who are not as physically able as others become further marginalised. Inevitably, the standards of sporting excellence and conceptions of the athletic bodies that are given most coverage and which are powerful in the process of socialisation are those of able-bodied, primarily male athletes. The bodies of impaired athletes are therefore continually judged in relation to an able-bodied 'norm', and the standards of play and performance are compared with those of mainstream competitions. As we have seen, however, certain classes of athletes – low-lesion paraplegics and leg amputees that can benefit from the improved technology that is a product of a normalising disability industry – are seen as being most worthy of media and sponsorship attention.

Developing this further, DePauw (1997) examines how sport marginalises the impaired and argues that we need to re-examine the relationship between sport and the body as it relates to disability:

> Ability is at the centre of sport and physical activity. Ability, as currently socially constructed, means 'able' and implies a finely tuned 'able' body. On the other hand, disability, also a social construction, is often viewed in relation to ability and is, then, most often defined as 'less than' ability, as not able. To be able to 'see' individuals with disabilities as athletes (regardless of the impairment) requires us to redefine athleticism and our view of the body, especially the 'sporting body'.
>
> (DePauw 1997: 423)

As a result of the focus on sporting performances, athletes that cannot perform in a manner that is considered 'normal' might be drawn to leisure activities where the body is not a central focus. Again, DePauw suggests

> It is through the study of the body in the context of, and in relation to, sport that we can understand sport as one of the sites for the reproduction of social inequality in its promotion of the traditional view of athletic

performance, masculinity, and physicality, including gendered images of the ideal physique and body beautiful.

(DePauw 1997: 420)

The marginalisation of the severely impaired body is exacerbated by the process of the distinct classification systems in place within sport for the disabled.

Marginalised by classification

The IPC has attempted to shift expectations and change the views of society in relation to people with a disability and athletes by presenting a 'normalised' view of sport for the disabled. Explicit attempts to streamline athletic classification are a product of this normalisation. As Chapter 4 suggests, the act of classification may be seen as a crucial mechanism for controlling sport for the disabled communitas, but it should also be seen as a means of controlling individual bodies. Closer alignment with the Olympic Movement has in part been responsible for the pressure to streamline classification systems by reducing the number of competitive categories available for participants. This shift has had a significant impact upon the elimination of classes and has particularly affected the more severely impaired athletes and events that are staged for women. One of the goals of the IOSDs is to champion the cause of just these groups, which already lack competitive opportunities (Howe and Jones 2006).

As a result of streamlining within the classification system, more severely impaired competitors are being marginalised within the Paralympic programme. Events for the more impaired athletes are excluded because often neither the event nor the athlete fits the image that is associated with athletic competitions or the ideal athletic body. These events are seen as less marketable and narrower in their appeal. These elite participants are being given sporting opportunities in events like boccia, which is removed from the environs of the athletics stadium and swimming pool that are the focus of most media attention during the Games. Boccia is a game of skill, similar to lawn bowls, played by athletes with severe cerebral palsy. In the context of the Paralympic Games, it is confined to indoor gymnasia. This shift away from the main stadiums where either swimming or athletics take place could imply that the competition in boccia is liminal to the larger spectacle of the Paralympic Games. The involvement of impaired performers in competitive sport is in effect accepting the social definitions of the importance of physical prowess – in essence disabling them (Hahn 1984).

I had hoped that this research would reveal a sense of communitas between elite impaired athletes – that is, a 'communion of equal individuals who submit together to the general authority of the ritual elders' (Turner 1969: 96). In this monograph the IPC can be seen as a form of ritual elder – and can institution to whom athletes must pay heed. Athletes with a disability are far more differentiated than a simple communitas, since they distinguish themselves by the degree of difference from the able-bodied norm and, as previously mentioned, established social relations on the back of a hierarchy of difference (Sherrill and Williams 1996: 48). Goffman, over forty years ago, stated:

> The more the child is 'handicapped' the more likely he is to be sent to a special school for persons of his kind, and the more abruptly he will have to face the view which the public at large take of him. He will be told that he will have an easier time of it among 'his own', and thus learn that the own he thought he possessed was the wrong one, and that this lesser own is really his.
>
> (Goffman 1963: 47)

In spite of the dated terminology, this statement is an accurate reflection of much that I have observed in relation to the marginalisation of differently classified bodied within Paralympic sport. Many of the athletes who were involved in the 1980s in sport for the disabled were the products of special schools, though most of the educational establishments were not just for one specific impairment group. As a result, the socialisation of these individuals was distinct from that of those who have impairments but are products of contemporary inclusive education. One fact remains the same: wherever the impaired are educated, their bodies marginalise them in relation to physical education. In special schools physical education adaptations are 'normal', but in the world of inclusive education today adaptations within sport actively 'other' impaired students, stigmatising them. This suggests that special schools may actually be advantageous for the recruitment of Paralympians, since greater numbers will be engaged in the practice of sport. Whether students at special schools are appropriately socialised in high-performance sport remains to be seen. Certainly many of my observations throughout the monograph from the mid- to late 1980s suggest the special school environment encourages participation but by and large steers clear of the fact that there is a possibility for students in their adult years to become high-performance athletes.

Many Paralympians become impaired later in life, so educational segregation does not affect them directly. However, they will be aware in part from the act of re-embodiment (Seymour 1998) that the Euro-centric rhetoric of integration and inclusion does little to ease the feelings of marginality associated with sporting practice.

Impaired bodies of athletes need to be classified in an equitable manner if the practice of the Paralympic Games is to function smoothly. Constant pressure to eliminate classes has an impact on athletes that is far greater than simply closing the door to Paralympic competition. For example, the removal of several classes from the athletics programme of the Paralympic Games is not considered negatively by the IPC, in the light of their mandate to reduce the number of classes; rather, it is seen as a necessary evil if the Games are to 'progress'. In spite of increased acceptance of sport for the disabled in society generally, the push to reduce the number of classification categories within sport for the disabled has had a dramatic effect on the people that should be central to its mission – the more severely impaired athletes. These athletes are being forced out of the sports, like track and field athletics, that are considered to be the 'shop window' of disability sport (Shogun 1998, 1999; Hughes 2000). For example, in 1988 there were lower class cerebral palsy athletes competing on the track, but by the mid-1990s athletes in this class were active only in field events. The nature of field events, where competitors are ultimately competing against their own performance, is such that the events themselves are seldom the centre of attention (such events are often staged in one corner of the infield while the track takes centre stage). Here, the body in a sense disappears. On the track, where an event by the very fact that it is in the centre of the stadium is centre stage, the aesthetics of these athletes' bodies can be vital to selling sponsorship and providing commercial opportunities.

This does, however, send the message that there are certain forms of physicality that are more acceptable (aesthetically pleasing) than others within the Paralympic Movement. In many respects the marginalisation of athletes with cerebral palsy within the sport of athletics is a case in point. Former CP-ISRA president Colin Rains stated:

> It's tough to say, but I believe people think that athletes with cerebral palsy are not totally media friendly, visually. They can be slightly uncoordinated both in their running and their visual expressions. It is possible people find this off-putting.
>
> (Mott 2000)

Hahn (1984) argues that by taking part in competitive sport, the disabled communitas is accepting the social definitions of the importance of physical prowess and, by doing so, underlining the inferior role of the disabled.

A more familiar association with impairments can be seen to be tied up with the concept of misfortune. Those athletes that appear to gain the most respect from the general public are those who have acquired their impairment through some form of accident. Within this group it is the least impaired, who can use technology to enhance their performance (see Chapter 7), that benefit the most from sport for the disabled generally and from the media spotlight associated with the Paralympic Games. If we look at the events that gain the majority of the attention on the international sporting stage, only lower spinal cord lesion impairments are part of the Olympic programme of athletics. It has been suggested by DePauw (1997) that it is society's view of athleticism and physicality that needs to be redefined if this situation is to change. On the other hand, it may have as much to do with the social construction of sporting objectivity. The objective parameter of time shows the wheelchair athletes are able to produce better times than able-bodied athletes over any distance longer than 800 m. While performances are continually improving for athletes who do not use technological aids (see Chapter 7), and more and more are adopting professional attitudes towards their training, they are unlikely ever to exceed the performances of the able-bodied elite. This will impact upon the opportunities for the non-cyborg athletes to attract media attention.

Research highlighting the deficiencies of television coverage during the 1996 Paralympic Games (Schell and Duncan 1999) and research concerning coverage in the print media in the United Kingdom (Thomas and Smith 2003; Smith and Thomas 2005) suggests there is a long way to go before equity is achieved in media coverage. It has been argued by DePauw (1997) that in spite of a lack of equity for the athlete with a disability, there has over time been a reduction in the degree to which athletes with an impairment have been marginalised. Such a decrease has taken some time but may be loosely seen in three steps:

The disabled have

1   been invisible or excluded from sport (invisibility of disability in sport)
2   become visible in sport as disabled athletes (visibility of disability in sport)
3   increasingly become visible in sports as athletes [(in) Visibility of disAbility in sport]

(DePauw 1997: 424)

Society today can be seen as attempting to enter the third phase of this progression, but, as the argument articulated throughout this monograph suggests, there is a considerable distance to travel before this aim is achieved. In fact, for the most severely impaired it could be argued that we are entering into a fourth phase where less visibility is being achieved. This is problematic, not least in terms of the values of Paralympism.

The removal of severely impaired sportspeople from the most visible venues at the Paralympic Games, such as the athletics track, would have come a lot sooner if calls from some quarters of the sport for the disabled to have the Paralympic Games integrated with the Olympic Games (Labonowich 1988) had been answered. This may have had the effect of improving media coverage of sport for the disabled but it would have come at the price of the severely impaired. It has been argued that the establishment of the IOSDs has had the effect of further institutionalising athletes with impairments so that they are not only marginalised from the mainstream but also from athletes from other groups who compete in sport. Such is the structure of sport for the disabled that the expression 'divide and conquer' might be an apt way of expressing the system that exists. Scholars such as Oliver (1990) have been suggesting that this is what the 'able' world wants, and it is no secret that the IOC forced the development of the IPC (Labonowich 1988) as a measure to secure the unavailability of disabled athletes for the Olympic Games. By established a performative environment separate to the Olympics, the athletes with imperfect bodies would not steal the media spotlight from the main event. Over time, however, those involved with the Paralympics at the performative end desired to be part of the elite sporting spectacle that is the Olympic Games, and there has been renewed pressure to push for integration, including involvement in full medal status events at the Commonwealth Games (Kalbfuss 2002; Smith and Thomas 2005).

Classification and performance-specific technology distinguishes sport for the disabled from that for the mainstream. However, in coverage by the media these two key features are seldom mentioned. Using content analysis, it has been determined that in Britain national print media the quantity of news coverage of disabled sport has increased since 1988, but there is little or no mention of classification in this 'improved' coverage. The big drawback of the classification system is the confusion it may cause, according to the former President of the IPC:

> Able-bodied classification is readily accessible and easy to understand, whereas classification of athletes with a disability involves a medical exam, requires an anatomical determination, is complicated, and is difficult to explain to the public.
>
> (Steadward 1996: 32)

It is important to realise the agenda behind such a statement. The IPC wants to reduce the number of classes to create a more media-friendly environment (Cole 1999). Issues of classification may not be exciting, and hence may be targets for the cutting room floor but it is paramount that the public who read about sport for the disabled are aware of the existence of such a system, since such an education would inevitable help public perception of sport for the impaired. Without this education-driven coverage, a lack of understanding of the variety of performances across impairment groups will confuse the public and diminish any sporting spectacle for the impaired.

Representation of athletes with disabilities in mainstream media may be conceived as leading eventually to the marginalisation of their 'otherness'. If this is to occur, media coverage surrounding the Paralympics must bond the distinctive sporting habitus and the sporting news. In 1984, intense media exposure of international sporting festivals transformed the Olympics from a sporting event into a mediated commercial sporting spectacle. For the Paralympic Movement, this shift began at the 1988 Paralympic Games in Seoul, South Korea (see Chapters 2 and 3).

In sport for the disabled, media attention has had the same impact as it has had on the transition and transformation of other sporting activities. A shift from pastime to spectacle has been well documented historically (Howe 2004a), and in the late twentieth century this transformation had begun to occur in the arena of sport for the disabled. The dilemma that this produces is that the general public's reticence regarding difference has meant a push by the IPC to get rid of lower disability classes, as they do not portray the 'proper' image of the elite athlete. The perception that certain Paralympic athletes should be taken seriously and others, in part because of the type of impairment they 'possess', should not, has made it difficult for national sporting organisations to effectively implement integrated sporting policy. For a specific example of this, we now look at the case of integration within Athletics Canada.

Integration and sport: the case of Athletics Canada

The integration process that is being undertaken by Sport Canada is seen as important if an inclusive society is to be achieved. Integration, broadly speaking, is the equal access for and acceptance of all in the communitas. Some scholars have distanced themselves from the discussion of integration, since the concept implies that the disabled population are required to change or be normalised in order to join the mainstream (Oliver 1996; Ravaud and Stiker 2001). In other words, the concept of integration requires members of the disabled communitas to adopt an 'able' disposition in order to become members of the mainstream. Yet scholars working within sports studies have adopted a continuum of integration that is useful in the current exploration of Athletics Canada. In their study of integration of sport for the disabled within the Norwegian sport system, Sørensen and Kahrs (2006) have adopted a continuum of compliance with the aim of exploring the success of their nation's inclusive sport system. Integration occurs when both the athletes with disabilities and the those from the mainstream adapt their cultural systems, and is referred to as *true* integration. Where athletes with a disability are forced to adopt the mainstream culture without any attempt at a reciprocal action, this is referred to as assimilation. Finally, the least integrated model is seen as segregation, where neither group is willing to transform its core cultural values in spite of being jointly managed within the sport system. This approach to understanding differing degrees of integration is, while somewhat arbitrary, useful when analysing the material that follows.

It is the process of true integration, which allows an inclusive society to be established, that is most relevant. If society is going to become more inclusive, 'it is necessary for existing economic, social and political institutions to be challenged and modified. This means that disabled people [*sic*] are not simply brought into society as it currently exists but rather that society is, in some ways, required to change' (Northway 1997: 165). True integration therefore has to be undertaken in order to establish an inclusive National Sports Organisation.

Bearing this in mind, scholars more recently have shown that integration can be effectively understood as an outcome (van de Ven *et al.* 2005) of an inclusive society. More specifically, it is argued that '[i]ntegration occurs through a process of interaction between a person with a disability and others in society' (van de Ven *et al.* 2005: 319). In other words, it is the process of interaction between an individual with a disability who possesses his or her own attitude toward integration, strategies and social roles, and others in society who adopt certain attitudes and images of people with disabilities. As a result, factors that influence the success of the integration process are both personal as well as social, but also include an element of support provision that will be distinct depending on the severity of the individual's disability (van de Ven *et al.* 2005; see also Kelly 2001).

It is possible, for example, to see true integration as a literal intermixing that entails the culture of both groups adapting to a new cultural environment. Dijker uses the term community integration to articulate a similar conceptualisation of true integration. Community integration as highlighted by Dijkers (1999: 41):

> is the acquiring of age, gender, and culture-appropriate roles, statuses and activities, including in(ter)dependence in decision making, and productive behaviours performed as part of multivariate relationships with family, friends, and others in natural community settings.

True integration therefore is 'a multifaceted and difficult process, which although it could be defined at a policy level rhetoric, [is] much less easy to define in reality' (Cole 2005: 341). The difficulty when exploring the success of integration policies is that the balance between the philosophical position and the reality (in this case a cultural sport environment) is not always clear. Simply exploring the policy landscape means that any interpretation is devoid of explicit cultural influences, though all policy is a cultural artefact. This being said, the aim of integration is to allow the disabled to take a full and active role within society. The ideal would be

> [a] world in which all human beings, regardless of impairment, age, gender, social class or minority ethnic status, can co-exist as equal members of the community, secure in the knowledge that their needs will be met and that their views will be recognised, respected and valued. It will be a very different world from the one in which we now live.
>
> (Oliver and Barnes 1998: 102)

Within the context of high-performance sport, this aim is hard to achieve. By its very nature, elite sport is selective and is based on how well individual bodies perform against one another (DePauw 1997). This can lead to individuals with or without disabilities being excluded (Bowen 2002). Determining the success of the integration process within Athletics Canada is not easy. As such, I would like to return to explore more fully the story of Chantel Petitclerc that was used in Chapter 1 to highlight the Paralympic 'coming of age'. Those who have read this monograph from cover to cover will be aware that the success of Petitclerc at the Sydney 2000 Paralympic Games does not illuminate the cultural politics behind the Paralympic Movement – the intervening material has been my attempt to shed light on the underbelly of the developments within sport for the disabled – but events following the next Games in Athens highlighted the distinction between sugar-coated media portrayals of 'heroism' and the reality of a lack of equality for high-performance athletes with an impairment.

Integration in action

Since the 2000 Paralympic Games, Petitclerc has been treated as a heroine by the Canadian press and applauded by the public as a role model for high-performance athletes across the country. In relation to other Canadian Paralympic champions she is in part the acceptable face of sport for the disabled – photogenic, charismatic, high functioning and an international winner. By the very nature of disabled sport, however, some athletes who are World and Paralympic Champions are excluded from the media spotlight often filled by the likes of Petitclerc. Petitclerc is a very able user of a wheelchair, and while she is one of the best within her classification, there are other Canadians who are also great champions but compete in different classes and who do not get the same degree of attention; as a result, issues and debates surrounding classification continue to be of concern (Seymour 1998; Wu and Williams 1999). The lack of equity of treatment of champions is just one issue facing Athletics Canada in its attempt to integrate athletes with a disability into its mainstream programmes.

The move to mainstream track and field athletics within Athletics Canada was preceded by the integration of the sport of swimming within the same framework in 1994. In 1997, high-performance wheelchair-user members of the Canadian Wheelchair Sports Association became part of Athletics Canada. The other national affiliates of the IOSDs, who all continue to be funded by Sport Canada, entered into negotiation with Athletics Canada to have their elite athletes integrated. By 2002, high-performance athletes who were the responsibility of the IOSDs were included officially within the framework of Athletics Canada, though they had become unofficial members of Athletics Canada while negotiations continued with the various disability sports organisations in the late 1990s.

The advent of a Paralympic manager within Athletics Canada in 1999 was facilitated in part because of Sport Canada's desire to see sports integrated across its programmes. At this stage, the role and responsibility of the manager was to liaise with Sport Canada primarily about funding (carding) for the athletes. The Athletes Assistance Program (AAP), which has in various forms been available to elite able-bodied athletes for several decades, was now available to Paralympians. This funding program is designed to offset some of the costs of training, but unless the athlete is supported by family members it does not facilitate full-time athlete status. Opportunities such as this within high-performance sport for the disabled, to be rewarded for the hours of hard work in the gym and on the track or field, represent a coming of age for Paralympic sport. The adoption of more comprehensive funding within Athletics Canada for athletes with a disability is also an important step in validating the identities of these people as high-performance athletes. To many within the Paralympic programme, acceptance within the mainstream able-bodied organisation is seen as justifying the hard work and energy put into their training by rewarding them with funding from Sport Canada.

The desire to organise a high-performance programme for Paralympic athletes separately within Athletics Canada suggests that true integration

(Sørensen and Kahrs 2006) is an issue that has not been properly tackled. There is a perception within the Paralympic programme that some athletes gain the benefits of carding and support from Athletics Canada while not having to work as hard as others, because the classification system advantages some impairment groups. A veteran of many Paralympic Games elaborates:

> It really does not seem fair that people such as them should get funding. I mean look at the physical state of [him]! Are we to believe that he has done the appropriate type of training? His gut is offensive. If I were to let myself go like that I would be nowhere near fit enough to make the team. What does it say about the depth of his class when he can get carded and be in such bad physical shape? To some of us the fact that [he] is part of the Athletics Canada programme makes a mockery of the term 'high performance'.

The issue highlighted above is of concern to a great many of the carded athletes. Carding should be a perk for those who train well. In essence, a carded athlete should see training as a full-time occupation, in spite of the fact that carding money, by itself, is not enough to sustain an individual with no family, friends or sponsors to rely on. If some athletes are not committed to training, achieving carded status becomes devalued. Another athlete expressed similar sentiments, but was clear about the differences between Paralympians.

> I do not care whether some athletes can win medals without training. It seems to me that if you are being funded by Sport Canada you have a responsibility to be as well trained as possible. I would say that at least a quarter of the team need to train harder. They simply haven't got the commitment that I think a high-performance athlete should have.

To many athletes, being carded reduces the financial burden of training. However, this carries an important responsibility. Receipt of the money necessarily imposes an obligation on the athlete to devote considerable time to training. In this respect, the athletes that are funded by Athletics Canada can be divided into those with a commitment to performing at their best, with all that entails, and those who are simply taking the money. Athletics Canada currently has forty AAP cards to give out to athletes on the Paralympic programme, and anything up to 20 per cent of these athletes are not training as effectively as they could be. This may be a direct result of many of the athletes being 'products' of the IOSD disability-specific system, where the participation ethos has been seen as more important than high-performance goals. A lack of communication between the national coaches that are part of the Paralympic programme and athletes might be exacerbated by the fact that Athletics Canada only looks after high-performance disabled athletes. While Athletics Canada maintains a degree of responsibility for grass-roots development in mainstream athletics (Green and Houlihan 2005), it has limited contact with potential athletes for the Paralympic programme. This can make talent identification problematic and if the Paralympic programme needs to card a certain number of athletes (or lose the funding) it will return to known athletes who may be a product the participation model of established by the IOSDs.

The image of an athlete with a disability who does not undertake training at the level expected of a high-performance athlete can have negative consequences for the organisation of Paralympic programmes. Structurally, the Paralympic programme at Athletics Canada is included within the provision of services for high-performance athletes, but it is clearly not truly integrated. The Paralympic programme manager with Athletics Canada has the responsibility to work alongside the paid head coach selecting the team of national coaches and the athletes for various international competitions. This leads to a situation where all Paralympic athletes are the responsibility of the Paralympic programme head coach and manager.

Athletics Canada is organised broadly into three event areas: endurance, speed and power, and Paralympic. In other words, an athlete with a disability who runs 5000 m is the responsibility of the Paralympic programme. If the Paralympic programme were truly integrated, the event areas might replace Paralympic with wheelchair racing, as the latter is distinctive to running. Profiled athletes on the organisation's webpage are also highlighted by their impairment group. By implication, a javelin thrower with cerebral palsy is not of the same status as his or her 'able' equivalent.

The status of the Paralympic programme within Athletics Canada is not currently a form of true integration. The Canadian public has largely been supportive of the integration process within their society. Chantel Petitclerc, who had a highly successful athletics season in 2004, winning the Olympic demonstration T54 wheelchair 800 m, followed up on this several weeks later at the Paralympic Games by breaking three World and one Paralympic record on the way to winning all five races she contested. The phenomenal form of Petitclerc on the track meant that the media spotlight intensified. At the end of this remarkable year she was honoured internationally at the sixth annual Laureus World Sports Awards as the best disabled athlete, by news magazine *Maclean's* as 'Canadian of the Year', and as by Canadian Women's magazine *Chatelaine* 'Women of the Year'.

Accommodation not integration

While the public in Canada celebrated Petitclerc's success there are still problems relating to the integration of Paralympic athletes into mainstream athletics. A lack of integration manifested itself in such a way that I believe that Sørensen and Kahrs' (2006) typology of integration, which can be seen as a continuum between true integration and exclusion, with assimilation occupying the middle ground, can be further expanded. Between assimilation and exclusion is where Athletics Canada's current integration model stands. This could be termed 'accommodation', because there is little acceptance within Athletics

Canada of the value associated with the Paralympic programme. Petitclerc's triumphant season of 2004 is a good example of this.

After victories on both the Olympic and the Paralympic stage, Petitclerc was 'honoured' at home by Athletics Canada, being jointly made 'Athlete of the Year'. Petitclerc refused to accept the award she was to share with 100m hurdler Perdita Felicien, a world-class athlete and world indoor champion who fell at the start of her final in Athens. Rejection of the award could be seen as a stance emblematic of the 'black power' salute famously given by Tommy Smith and John Carlos during the medal ceremony for the 200m during the Mexico Olympic Games in 1968, since in essence Petitclerc was standing up not only for her own achievement but also for those of all elite athletes with a disability in the nation.

Athletics Canada may have been acting appropriately by nominating both an able and a disabled athlete for the award, but Petitclerc saw it as a snub. She said of the award,

> To me, it's really a symptom that [Athletics Canada] can't evaluate the value of a Paralympic medal – that it's easier to win a Paralympic medal than an Olympic medal. That may have been true 15 years ago. That's not the case any more.
>
> (Wong 2004)

In the events in which Petitclerc competes, the depth of the field is as great as any in able-bodied athletics. At the Olympic Games and other mainstream track and field athletics events, there is only ever a handful of likely winners of the top prize. The only difference is that at the Paralympic Games, particularly in events like wheelchair racing, the winners are drawn from nations that are often the most technologically advanced (see Chapter 7). While African athletes dominate middle-distance running at the Olympics, IAAF World Championships and Grand Prix circuit, the need for technology in wheelchair racing means that the winners are typically drawn from Westernised nations. The problem, according to Patrick Jarvis, former President of the Canadian Paralympic Committee and one of the few former Paralympians in a position of significant power within the Movement, is that

> We get many supportive comments as Paralympians. But as soon as you start to incur in their [able-bodied athletes] territory, being respected just as equal athletes and you threaten to win some of their awards, a lot are still uncomfortable with [disability].
>
> (Christie 2004)

If the shoe had been on the other foot and Felicien had won her race and Petitclerc had not won all she contested, would the honour have gone to both athletes? Presumably not. Clearly Peticlerc's actions suggested that she felt discriminated against. The Canadian Charter of Rights and Freedoms of 1982 includes disability as a prohibited ground for discrimination, and therefore she might feel rightfully aggrieved. It is no wonder that high-performance athletes with a disability are still today having difficulty with being integrated into mainstream sport.

Athletics Canada is not alone in paying little attention to the importance of integration. In spite of being at the forefront of human rights legislation regarding discrimination on the grounds of disability, true integration at all levels of sport is not happening. On 25 November 2003, the Canadian Secretary of State for Physical Activity in Sport, Paul DeVillers, announced the creation of a working group to examine the issues related to sport and disability. If Sport Canada is working as it should, why has such a group been launched over two decades after it was illegal to discriminate against people with a disability in Canada? Perhaps the following statement, made by an Athletics Canada official during an international event in 2005, highlights the struggle that the Paralympic programme faces – 'You guys are almost as serious as the able-bodied program'.

To the outsider, the integration of Paralympic Athletes within the matrix of Athletics Canada may be seen as a statement of a progressive nation. Nevertheless, integration within Athletics Canada has not been complete and, as a result heightens the social division between the able and the disabled within high-performance sport in Canada. While Athletics Canada has attempted to integrate athletes with a disability by branding them as products of their organisation, such gestures have done little to address the inequities within the organisations that favour the 'able' athletes. The process of accommodating the Paralympic Athletics programme within Athletics Canada has been relatively successful; however, integration or the intermixing of persons previously segregated has not. As Zola suggests,

> only when we acknowledge the near universality of disability and that all its dimensions (including the biomedical) are part of the social process by which the meanings of disability are negotiated, will it be possible fully to appreciate how general public policy can affect this issue.
>
> (Zola 1989: 420)

Summary

Impairment is one of life's certainties. For those classed as impaired, it might be any form of physical or sensory task that marks us out as distinctive to the able; it may be any manner of activity – physical or otherwise. The distinction between those who are normal and those who are abnormal is relatively small, but the practice of sport and its reliance upon physical capital magnifies this difference. As Seymour suggests,

> It is undeniable that sport and physical activities provide a context for enjoyment, self-identity and competence, but unless the conditions and

ideology of sport are challenged, women, and indeed many men, will continue to operate in a context that compounds their disadvantage.

(Seymour 1998: 126)

This final chapter in this monograph is not a conclusion, but I hope a part of a growing literature that more than anything tackles the process of supercripisation. Having spent over twenty years living and researching this volume my particular anthropological lens is still focused upon the Paralympic Movement with a desire to illuminate the relationship between high-performance sport, the body and impairment. The end product is a contribution to the ongoing debate surrounding physicality and sporting practice. Each reader brings to his or her engagement with this text distinctive cultural baggage, and no doubt some will bring insight that, not for lack of trying, I will never have. There is a need to move away from the view adopted by the media that sport for the disabled is simply a virtuous practice, and engage with it as a practice that is as flawed as any other. Empowerment for the most impaired athletes is still a dream. By questioning the validity of the practice of sport for the disabled, we will at least make inroads into treating the impaired as normal.

Appendix
Through an anthropological lens

This appendix is not intended to be a how-to guide to ethnographic methodology, as other books provide informed and comprehensive accounts (see Bernard 1995; Hammersley and Atkinson 1995; Davies 1997); rather, its purpose is twofold. First, it forms a backdrop for engaging with some of the debates about representation within the social sciences, and anthropology specifically. Recent debate surrounding writing culture (Clifford and Marcus 1986; James *et al.* 1997; Coffey 1999; Davies 1997; Sparkes 2002) has drawn attention to the shortcomings of ethnographic methods. To a point these debates have validity, in that attempting to establish a concrete truth as a goal within the social sciences is a 'fool's errand'. The second aim of this appendix is to enable the reader to get a sense of my academic perspective and to suggest that, ultimately, social research into communities such as the IPC generally and the sport of track and field athletics for athletes with a disability specifically that adopts the methodology of ethnography can be fruitful. Because of this belief – in part bestowed on me through my training in anthropology, where to use methods other than participant observation was contrary to recent history of the discipline – this appendix will highlight the tensions of representation and issues of access before highlighting some of the ethnographic research that has been conducted on sporting contexts to great effect. The appendix should be seen as a useful guide in understanding the position of the author as the anthropologist at the centre of the research, and this, along with the details of how I happened to become involved in the Paralympic community (see Chapter 1), should give the reader a sense of my position in the field and an understanding of the 'authority', though wholly culturally constructed, with which I speak on the Paralympic Movement.

Ethnography: a brief history of its use and key debates

In recent years ethnography has become a popular approach to the social investigation of sporting cultures. There is, however, some confusion as to what constitutes the use of ethnographic methods within the multi-disciplinary field of sports studies. The term 'ethnography' is used in two distinct ways within social research: for ethnographic research and for an ethnographic monograph. It does not mean simply 'qualitative'. As a noun, it means a description of a culture, or a piece of a culture. As a verb (doing ethnography), it means the collection of data that describes a culture. It is simply a methodology of social scientific research. Ethnography is characterised by the first-hand study of a small community or ethnic group. This form of study combines varying degrees of descriptive and analytical elements, but of key importance in conventional ethnographies is that they focus on one specific culture or society and consider theoretical or comparative generalisations from the standpoint of the ethnographic example.

The history of participant observation as part of the ethnographic tool-kit is rather unclear, since the act of performing this type of research is closely linked with the way that people make sense of their worlds on a daily basis. The origin of the modern ethnographic research tradition is generally traced to Bronislaw Malinowski (1884–1942) in the field of anthropology, or the rise of the Chicago School in sociology, where the primacy of field research and participant observation was stressed. Participant observation, the act of living within and being involved with a community, is at the heart of traditional ethnographic practice, but is only one of many tools employed by the ethnographer. A researcher using the ethnographic tool kit will, as well as participating and observing the community in question, undertake research in the library, develop and employ survey techniques and structured and semi-structured interviews, and record natural conversations as a way of illuminating a cultural environment.

Ethnography from the post-war period until recently had acquired a generally ahistorical perspective, concentrating on the reconstruction of a specific cultural or social system without regard to its historical development, and relegating historical considerations to a separate area labelled as the 'study of social cultural change', as if this were at odds with normal features of historical groups. A related feature of this type of ethnography is the tendency artificially to isolate the unit of study (the tribe, the peasant community etc.), considering it as a self-contained culture or society and failing to take into account regional, national and international politico-economic and social structures with which the local community interacts. This tendency in conventional ethnography has been amply criticised from many directions by those that have sought to establish a new type of ethnography which is conscious of both the historical process and multi-layered power structures as these impinge on the community under investigation.

To confuse matters, ethnographers refer to participant observation as 'fieldwork'. Fieldwork therefore is synonymous with the collection of data using observational methods. The making, reporting and evaluation of these observations is the task of the ethnographer. In order to be meaningful, the observations should be related to interpretation derived from the socio-cultural imagination. Good ethnography attempts to avoid overt ethnocentrism – that is, the habit or tendency to judge other cultures (or communities under investigation) according to the criteria of the ethnographers' own culture.

Participant observation, or ethnographic fieldwork, is the foundation of cultural anthropology. It involves getting close to people and making them feel comfortable enough with your presence so that you can observe and record information about their lives.

(Bernard 1995: 137)

Simply put, this involves establishing a rapport in the social environment that is under investigation, and a pattern so that you are as unobtrusive as possible while members of the community are going about their daily lives. A degree of skill is required to achieve these aims and to avoid complete cultural immersion, so that you can make detailed notes about the events of the day. In time you will be able to turn to these data, put your cultural experience into perspective and articulate this in a written form. In other words,

The participant observer gathers data by participating in the daily life of the group or organisation he studies. He watches the people he is studying to see what situations they ordinarily meet and how they behave in them. He enters into conversation with some or all of the participants in these situations and discovers their interpretations of the events he has observed.

(Becker 1958: 652)

Research using participant observation, then, means that the researcher is in the front line as the main instrument of social investigation. This methodological approach allows for the collection of data on any number of things, including social interactions in real time. Ethnographic fieldwork is most successful when numerous methods are used within the same social environment.

As 'participant observation', fieldwork is an experience as well as a method, but it is emphatically method and not just experience. The main instrument of this method is the fieldworkers themselves, but they must struggle to harness their subjectivity towards the purpose of the research, which is an understanding of human experience that is somewhat systematic and objective – more so, at least, than a casual impression or common sense. Nothing is less useful than an adventure without meaning, an encounter without notes, and much of the data of fieldwork comes through rather tedious observations and recording. The deepest insights may derive from a flash of understanding that comes from engagement and encounter. As the term 'participant observation' suggests, fieldwork combines objectivity and subjectivity, routine and adventure, system and openness.

Bernard (1995) has suggested that there are two roles within fieldwork – the participating observer and the observing participant – while others have suggested there are four – those mentioned by Bernard as well as the complete observer and the complete participant (Burgess 1984; Hammersley and Atkinson 1995). The role of the complete participant can provide data that is less diluted than the other roles, because the community under investigation is unaware of the researcher's involvement in the project. As such, the data have not been shaped by the informants knowing that they were informants; however, it also means that the researcher is presented with an ethical dilemma, such as whether it is appropriate to adopt a covert role in the aid of any research project. As a result, most authoritative sources regarding how to conduct this type of research have a section on ethical considerations (see Hammersley and Atkinson 1995).

Though based on fieldwork, ethnography is also a way of generalising about humanity. Like the novel, poem and parable, but also like the scientific experiment, ethnography must say more than it tells; it must imply and teach general significances through presentation of particular experiences and patterns. Among the 'truths' communicated are the ethnographer's as well as the native's, yet few care to read the confessional memoirs of an ethnographer. A great ethnographic work is both scientific and literary, attaining a marked degree of objective precision, yet translating patterns discerned in the alien group into a form comprehensible to the reader at home (see Armstrong 1998; Klein 1993).

This has changed for some scholars in recent years, and there has been a trend toward the use of autobiography (Davies 1997) or what has been called 'auto-ethnography' (Sparkes 2002). This is relevant on a number of levels. First, autobiography allows ethnographers to realise that their data are the product of a social world of which they as interpreter are a key element. On another level of interest is the experience of fieldwork of ethnographers. which is key to the interpretations they make in the field. This is not dissimilar to auto-ethnography. Auto-ethnography is distinct because the self is the central vehicle for understanding the social world. The world of the ethnographer is what is being explored. Where traditionally the 'truths' of the interpretation, filtered through the experience and worldview of the interpreter but focused sharply and precisely on the world of the 'other', is the focus of ethnography, auto-ethnography is concerned largely with the position of the researcher in the world. The danger of this phenomenological position is that the truths discerned by self-examination may be too closely bound to the experience of the researcher and the categories of their culture.

Although ethnography has undoubtedly enhanced the understanding of sporting cultures and communities, it is an approach that has been subject to critique from within and without anthropology. Notably, the traditional view within anthropology of an objective social science has been brought into question, leading to a 'crisis of representation' within the discipline and elsewhere in the social sciences (Clifford and Marcus 1986; Marcus and Fischer 1986). This crisis

> alerted anthropologists to the need to pay closer attention to the epistemological grounds of their representations and, furthermore, has made them consider the practical import of that process of reflection, both for the anthropological endeavour and for those who are the subjects of any anthropological enquiry.
>
> (James *et al.* 1997: 3)

In a sense, then, the postmodern turn in anthropology (Clifford and Marcus 1986; Marcus and Fischer 1986) and in the social sciences more generally (Coffey 1999) has led to a discussion about the validity of ethnographic methods. The bottom line in many of these debates is simply that 'objectivity is impossible' and 'subjectivity undesirable' (Peacock 1986: 87). Doing ethnography, these debates suggest, is not as simple as going on holiday and writing a diary, because the act of participant observation is trapped in a cultural environment that is continually being transformed not just by the peoples being researched but also by the researcher (Clifford 1986). The product of the ethnographer – the literary output, whether fieldnotes, draft or published texts from the research – is steeped in a distinctive cultural heritage. As a result, '[e]thnographic truths are thus inherently *partial* – committed and incomplete' (Clifford 1986: 7).

Given the complexity of ethnography, it is obviously difficult to generalise globally based on single ethnographic accounts. It is wrong to synthesise merely substantive or 'factual' findings of ethnographic investigations, for each ethnography is more than a report, a mere shortcut for being there. Each is an interpretation, a synthesis of questions, theories and attitudes that guide the interpreter, as well as facts reported. At the same time, the empirical or inductive approach characteristic of social scientific generalisation is a necessary antidote to purely deductive or introspective efforts at reflecting on human nature.

Some researchers have argued that in situations where there is a risk involved in telling your informants the reason you are present, such action might be justified. In the case of sports ethnography, the work of Armstrong (1998) on football hooligans in Sheffield, and that of Sugden and Tomlinson on the use of investigative journalism to explore ticket touts in the game of world football (Sugden and Tomlinson 1999), also required a degree of risk that was not required in order to undertake research on the Paralympic Movement. In both of these cases the researchers felt that the use of degrees of covert methods of participant observation were a necessity to provide a safe environment in which to undertake their research. When it comes to issues of representation, however, it should not be assumed that because the research was undertaken in a covert manner the presence of the researcher does not alter the research environment, because any interaction with the community will have an impact on the recorded data. There is also a possibility that the researcher can be handicapped by the assumed role within the group (Burgess 1984), making it more difficult to gather data – the primary reason for being with the group in the first place. In the extreme the researcher might 'go native', which means he or she stops recording data altogether and begins to live a normal life within the community. When ethnographic methods were used on 'exotic' peoples in faraway lands, it seems reasonable that going native would have been more difficult than in the social settings in which contemporary ethnographers often engage, which are located in more accessible Western contexts. In other words, going 'native' might hark back to the days of imperial anthropology, but it is more likely to occur within the tradition of ethnography in sociology known as the Chicago School, which more often than not focuses upon field sites that are not entirely culturally distinct from the researchers own background. Going native is distinct from experiential ethnography (Sands 2002: 126), since the latter has as its hallmark almost complete immersion, much the same as the former, but social distance behind the scenes is created through the act and art of writing down detailed observations. The fear of going native is real (and must be considered only a bad thing if completion of research the ultimate goal – it is not a bad thing in and of itself), and as a result ethnographic-based method texts suggest regular breaks from the 'field' in order to write up and reflect upon the experience of being a participant observer (Bernard 1995; Hammersley and Atkinson 1995).

The role of the participating observer as well as the observing participant facilitates an opportunity to collect much more detailed data, since being in these roles allows for the collection of data on a number of fronts. Such social distance facilitates the collection of data that ultimately can lead to a thick description of a social cultural environment that is predicated on the collection of detailed field notes (Geertz 1973). These notes are intended to be their author's representation of the social world under investigation. A key consideration is that the social world under investigation is a natural setting. Ethnographers traditionally chronicle the social world under investigation based on various accounts that they obtain from members of the community under investigation and from observations taken. By piecing together the social world according to various informants the collection of data becomes more comprehensive, and this is married with the theoretical insights developed as a result of the theory 'employed' to make sense of the world. This type of research, as highlighted in this monograph, leaves the ethnographer at risk of making claims about power relations that may be errant. Smith suggests:

> working in fieldsites where they are constantly made aware of the ways in which currently prevailing and historical fields of power give shape to a particular set of cultural meanings and practices, anthropologists run the risk of highlighting the *effects* of hegemonic processes through time, over and above the practices of identifiable agents with self-conscious hegemonic projects.
>
> (Smith 1999: 252)

It is of course important to realise that because the interaction (in the case of participant observation research) is face to face, the ethnographer has a role to play in shaping the social world under investigation. It is difficult if not impossible to know how the involvement of the ethnographer shapes the social environment, but what is certain is that in more long-term or diachronic studies of communities where the researcher is seen to be an adjunct member of the community the influence may be less marked. Today a community is not always the bounded entity that anthropologists engaged with in the past, such as a well-defined group of islanders living in remote regions. Rather, communities are more emotive than this. Recently, Amit (2002: 18) has suggested:

The emotive impact of community, the capacity for empathy and affinity, arise not just out of an imagined community, but in the dynamic inter-action between that concept and the actual and limited social relations and practices through which it is realized.

The nature of communities that are no longer seen as bounded means that most sport ethnography makes it more difficult for the ethnographer to make the dis-tinction between inside and outside of the research field. As such, unbounded communities can facilitate a transformation of the ethnographers' worldview to the point in some cases where they can find it difficult to distinguish the uniqueness of the cultural environment at the heart of the study. In many respects, then, the act of going native is not clear cut, but, in the context of anthropological literature, going native is often seen as a failing on behalf of ethnographers to position themselves in relation to the data they are investigat-ing – to become outright participants – more than simply engaging with the experience to the point where they fail to record observations. It is of course very difficult to balance the amount of participation and observation that the ethnographer is engaged in at any one time during the research process. However, the reflexive character of this form of social research implies

> that the orientations of researchers will be shaped by their socio-historical locations, including the values and interests that these locations confer upon them. What this represents is a rejection of the idea that social research is, or can be, carried out in some autonomous realm that is insu-lated from the wider society and the particular biography of the researcher, in such a way that its findings can be unaffected by the social processes and personal characteristics.
>
> (Hammersley and Atkinson 1995: 16)

Because of the issues and concerns highlighted above, and the fact that people who are members of the communities that social scientists wish to investigate, are not naive about the 'outsider' and the impact they may have on the social environment they are studying, issues of access are important. To many, enter-ing the field or gaining access to the field might be the most problematic part of ethnographic fieldwork (Bernard 1995).

Access to the field

Issues of access often vary depending on the ethnographer's cultural compe-tence in the community that is the target of the research project. The greater the level of cultural understanding, the less likely it is that the ethnographer will need to 'employ' numerous gatekeepers. Gatekeepers are quite simply the actors that control access to informants and the opportunities to meet a wide range of them during the fieldwork. These individuals then can be a catalyst to a successful or unsuccessful time in the field. Gatekeepers can be influential in the establishment of the legitimacy of the ethnographer, and as a result it is apparent that the data collected can be shaped as much by the gatekeepers, and their degree of access in the community as by the autobiography of the researcher. Peacock has suggested that entry into the field is a three-step process (Peacock 1986). In the first instance, the researcher needs to gain the experience in order to get there. This can take the form of training that is implicit in undergraduate fields of the social sciences, particularly anthropology, where, certainly in the mid-1980s, there was little explicit discussion about methods of research. Students simply read numerous ethnographic monographs and began to get a flavour of what was required to undertake this type of research. The second stage of fieldwork is to establish an identity in the community under investigation.

When a researcher goes into a community for the first time it is often difficult to become an outright participant, and in most cases ethnographers will at least need to engage in observing their new surroundings in order to establish where they might fit in, with the ultimate aim being to gain access to as many aspects of the community as possible. Developing a relationship with numerous gatekeepers and/or numerous points of entry into the social world surrounding the community is the third step of the entry process as highlighted by Peacock (1986). The idea is to gain insight into the particular cultural environment and to use the distinctive anthropological lens that we each possess. As I mentioned in Chapter 1, my access to the field of study in this monograph was my body. Being born with cerebral palsy allowed me access to sport for the disabled as an athlete. Over the years, I have established relationships with individual gatekeepers in the Paralympic communitas that have helped in shaping the outcomes of this research. The fact that I have taken on numerous roles within the IPC world has also helped in gaining appropriate access.

It should be made clear at this point that entry into the 'field' is neither clear cut nor simple, because the sites of ethnographic research are no longer demarcated distinctive environments (Marcus and Fischer 1986). Traditionally the understanding has been that an ethnographer is immersed in the field, establishes relationships with relevant gatekeepers, and simply extracts the data that provide a detailed cultural understanding. However, '[t]he notion of immersion implies that the "field" which ethnographers enter exists as an independently bounded set of relationships and activities which is autonomous of the fieldwork through which it is discovered' (Amit 2000: 6). Access to the field in many cases needs to be continually re-negotiated. Since the location of field sites is fluid, it makes access more problematic than in traditional community-based ethnography. In a sense, then, there has been a shift away from the place or location as the focal point for the development of culture. As Amit (2000: 13) suggests,

> The shift away from locality as the boundary and site for cultural production has allowed anthropologists to take more cognizance of migrants and travellers whose social networks and frames of reference are likely to be dispersed and multilocale rather than conveniently fixed in one place.

In light of this it seems that it is appropriate to explore the cultural politics of the Paralympic Movement where ethnographic data have been collected on various continents in a diachronic fashion over two decades. Following Appadurai (1991: 196),

> What a new style of ethnography can do is to capture the impact of deterritorialization on the imaginative resources of lived, local experiences. Put another way, the task for ethnography now becomes the unravelling of a conundrum: what is the nature of locality, *as lived experience*, in a globalizing, deterritorialized world?

Ethnographies of sport

Anthropology has been rather slow to embrace the need to examine the social milieu surrounding sport. The importance placed on the utilitarian nature of culture in traditional anthropology, as opposed to the expressive dimensions of culture, of which sport is a part, may help to explain this absence (Chick 1998). While early work by anthropologists such as Tylor (1896), Firth (1931) and Lesser (1933) examined the importance of sport in the social world, few have followed in their footsteps. Anthropologists such as Geertz (1973) and Foley (1990) have used the anthropological lens to examine sport, although sport was not their prime focus. The history of the anthropology of sport (see Blanchard 1995, Sands 1999a) is rather limited, but the adoption of ethnography as a cross-disciplinary methodological tool for furthering our understanding of the sporting world should be seen as a major contribution by anthropology to social research regarding sport. The related discipline of sociology has increasingly been the focus of high-quality research into the social environment surrounding sport (Ingham and Donnelly 1997), some of which has adopted the ethnographic method.

Over the past decade there has been an increase in the use of participant observation as a primary ethnographic tool for detailing sporting communities. Important ethnographic studies have been produced by anthropologists such as Armstrong (1998) on football hooligans, Foley (1990) on American football, Klein (1991, 1993) on baseball and bodybuilding, as well as several collections in the form of edited volumes (MacClancy 1996; Armstrong and Giulianotti 1997; Sands 1999b). Meanwhile, the recent work by Wheaton (1997, 2000) and Wheaton and Tomlinson (1998) on wind-surfing, by Sugden (1996) and by Mennesson (2000) on men's and women's boxing respectively, and by Blackshaw and Crabbe (2005) on 'deviance' are excellent examples of how non-anthropologists have embraced ethnography and put it to constructive use in describing and understanding the functioning of sporting cultures and in chronicling the transformation of these cultures. Others have argued that the use of autoethnography can facilitate a fruitful landscape of social cultural research. '[F]or the author comes the possibility of first recognising entrenched cultural narratives and dominant "master" narratives, and then rejecting them by writing in ways that both resist and challenge the accepted norm' (Sparkes 2002: 98). This said, by and large these auto-ethnographies are only capturing the narratives of those with the cultural capital to gain access to publishing outlets. As a result of the 'writing culture' debate highlighted above, auto-ethnography seems to be overtly introspective because it is simply passing on ethnographers' understandings of themselves. Other modern approaches to the art of interpreting the 'other' are still paramount to a robust ethnographic agenda (Sugden and Tomlinson 1999; Blackshaw and Crabbe 2005).

Those adopting ethnography as a research tool therefore became more sensitive to their own identity and the impact of this on their research findings. de Garis (1999) has gone so far as to suggest that the ethnography of sport should be turned into a sensuous ethnography where the participant ethnographer records all aspects of the sensuous experience of fieldwork. This new enlightened approach to ethnographic representation, coupled with other methodologies that are more commonly employed in social investigations of the sport (interview and survey), leads to a more complete understanding of the sporting world. The value of this type of data should not be underestimated and, contrary to suggestions by anthropologists such as Sands (1999c), these data have an equal role to play in constructing 'social reality' to the data collected by the use of the ethnographic method.

The investigative approach to sociological inquiry blends ethnography with investigative journalism, and with it a distinctive mix of skills for developing social distance in order to make sense of the research environment (Sugden and Tomlinson 1999). Sugden and Tomlinson (1999), borrowing from Ward (1999), advocate the use of an associational epistemology. This enables researchers to increase their understanding because of this approach's need for a moral imperative to be systematically rigorous as well as objective. Investigative sociologists who adopt ethnographic methods 'should have a commitment to the objective, rigorous and systematic quest for a socially constructed truth' (Sugden 2005: 206). Truth in this sense is sociological, de facto what passes for truth in the social world, and this is achieved by gaining access to as many social vantage points as possible.

In a recent book on deviance in sport, Blackshaw and Crabbe (2005) pointed out that the epistemology engaged in by Sugden and Tomlinson (1999) fails to place value on the understanding of surface meaning within a social situation; rather it appears that only 'deep' understanding or insight into the cultural milieu are of value. While the point raised by Blackshaw and Crabbe does have validity, bringing this well-placed objection to the attention of other ethnographers and students of sport studies, they fail to address an alternative or bridge the gap between deep and surface understandings of cultural worlds. This lacuna could neatly be addressed by suggesting an approach to observation that is based upon a 'thick description' regardless of where the observation took place – deep – away from the public eye or surface – open to view.

> What the ethnographer is in fact faced with ... is a multiplicity of complex conceptual structures, many of them superimposed upon or knotted into

one another, which are at once strange, irregular, and inexplicit, and which he must contrive somehow first to grasp and then to render.

(Geertz 1973: 10)

It is important, therefore, for the readers of this monograph to remember the points above as they reflect upon the text. In the chapters of this monograph, particularly those that focus on the contemporary world of the Paralympic Movement, the reader needs to bear in mind the cultural baggage (specifically highlighted in Chapter 1) which accompanies me as I peer through my anthropological lens. The self changes and transforms beside (and sometimes along with) the social environment under investigation and by its very nature then the act of construction of an ethnographic account is autobiographical: 'Fieldwork is personal, emotional and identity *work*' (Coffey 1999: 1). Yet it is not an exact reflection of the lived experience of the author, since

[t]he writing and reading of ethnography are overdetermined by forces ultimately beyond the control of either an author or an interpretive community. These contingencies – of language, rhetoric, power and history – must now be openly confronted in the process of writing.

(Clifford 1986: 25)

Summary

In a sense, my tactics for undertaking this research highlight the 'inextricable relationship between epistemology, politics and practice which the "Writing Culture" debate drew attention to' (James *et al.* 1997: 2). As such, an understanding of the fluidity of culture is key and important. We now know that

'Cultures' do not hold still for their portraits. Attempts to make them do so always involve simplification and exclusion, selection of a temporal focus, the construction of a particular self–other relationship, and the imposition or negotiation of a power relationship.

(Clifford 1986: 10)

The 'writing culture' debate surrounding issues of representation does provide insight to ethnographers, and is in fact one of the reasons this appendix was included in this monograph. It is important that readers know where the author is coming from – in other words, what methodological position I have taken in the field, combined with the autobiographical account of 'where I am coming from' and my observations about the Paralympics Movement (see Chapter 1), facilitates an insight into how data were collected.

Ultimately our daily task, whatever our role in life, is continually to re-evaluate the social world around us so that it continues to make sense. Largely, we do this unthinkingly. Our existence and the roles that we play are generally not questioned. It is apposite at this moment in time that those who occupy roles within the Paralympic Movement, regardless of how central those might be, examine whether their position enhances the opportunities of the practice community. As an indigenous ethnographer in the world of the Paralympic Movement, my embodiment enables an access to the inner sanctum of the culture that I am hopeful readers will have found enriching.

Notes

1 Athlete as anthropologist, anthropologist as athlete

1 Following the work of Victor Turner (1969: 96), the term 'communitas' is used throughout this volume to articulate the modality of social relations rather than an area of common living that the term community distinguishes.
2 This is a pseudonym for a weekly track and field athletics publication.
3 Cerebral palsy is often referred to simply by the acronym CP and, as such, throughout this volume either the full or the shortened form will be used.
4 This is a federation that was launched in September 2004 at the Athens Paralympic Games. It is the result of a merger of two federations, the International Stoke Mandeville Wheelchair Sports Federation (ISMWSF) and the International Sport Organisation for the Disabled (ISOD), that have been part of the Paralympic Movement since its inception. The launch of this new federation during the Athens Paralympic Games was greeted from some quarters as if it were the second coming of the IPC. The vast majority of power-brokers with the sport for the disabled have come from the antecedents of this new federation, and there was concern expressed by the other IOSDs that they might be squeezed out of the processes of decision-making.
5 *Sydney Morning Herald*, 23 October 2000.

2 A social history of sport for the disabled

1 The use of the word 'confined' is purposeful here, as this was the rhetoric that would have been seen as appropriate at the time
2 In 1924, the first IOSD was formed for athletes with a hearing impairment. Comité International des Sports Sourds (CISS) was a founding member of the IPC, but left in 1995. Because it is currently not a member of IPC and no hearing-impaired athletes (other than those with multiple impairments who are part of the other organisations) have competed in the Paralympic Games, this organisation is not considered of great importance in the discussion that follows.
3 http://www.paralympic.org/release/Main_Sections_Menu/IPC/About_the_IPC/ (retrieved 26 September 2007).
4 www.paralympic.org
5 This literally translates from the French as 'the others'. People with impairments that impacted on the body's function in the same manner as an amputation were allowed to compete.
6 INAS-FMH changed its name to the International Sports Federation for Persons with Intellectual Disabilities, or INAS-FID.
7 Webcasting is the showing of live competition through the Internet.
8 T54 is an event classification; the 'T' says that this is a track event, the '5' says that it

is an event for a wheelchair athlete, and the '4' means that the athlete is a highly mobile user of a wheelchair.

9 www.asianparalympic.org/aboutus/default.asp?action=profile (last accessed 20 April 2007)

3 Paralympic 'lived history': reflections of a participant observer

1 The structure of the IPC is constantly being transformed to move with the times. There currently is an athletes' committee, but it has very little real power. For a detailed look at the current structure consult the IPC website at www.paralympic.org.

2 This is a statement that has been made at every closing ceremony that I have attended. In the case of Barcelona I still believe the statement to be true, as no summer Paralympic Games has surpassed it – though it must be said I attended the Athens 2004 Games as a journalist so my point of view might be altered by these circumstances.

3 In other sports, such as swimming, it is two ... and each international sporting federations have different criteria.

4 For an interesting early discussion of this debate, see BBC (1994)

5 The IPC constitution only allows executive members to be in post for three four-year terms. Dr Bob Steadward was the IPCs first President, and was in office from 1989 until 2001.

6 The development of specialist *ad hoc* committees, such as those for the severely impaired and women, from the outside at least suggested that the IPC's policies targeting both groups that should be implemented by all in the IPC network were less than effective.

7 The IPCAC structure was transformed in 2006. From 2007 the Committee has been run by the IPC Athletics Sports Manager (a full-time employee of the IPC) and an appointed technical committee.

8 For a description of classification as it relates to track and field athletics, visit the IPCAC website at www.ipc-athletics.org.

9 www.paralympic.org

10 For reasons expressed in the introduction I prefer the term 'impairment', though the IPC uses the term 'disability'. Put simply, disability implies a social component to the situation of the person defined as such, whereas impairment is more directly concerned with the embodiment of the condition.

4 The politics of sporting disablement

1 See Andrews (1993) for an excellent review of Foucault's genealogy.

2 There is a tendency in mainstream sport to 'award' elite status to those who achieve the most in terms of physical performance. This is also to some degree the case within sport for the disabled, where certain types of disability lead to the assumption of non-elite status. As far as I was concerned, my status as an elite athlete was related to the commitment in training my body in the pursuit of excellence. In this way, by comparing the quality and quantity of training an athlete has undergone to achieve their best performance, a reasonable barometer on 'elite' status can be illuminated.

3 In some federations the classification team is different. The Cerebral Palsy International Sport Recreation Association (CP-ISRA) requires a medical doctor, a sports technical official and a physiotherapist, where as the International Blind Sports Federation (IBSA) only requires the services of certified ophthalmologist.

4 Those swimmers with visual impairment are not part of this system and compete using the IBSA classification system, details of which can be found at www.paralympic.org.

5 Most of these also required the timetabling of heats within the stadium.

6 The rules on competitiveness that eliminated the cerebral palsy male wheelchair

racers from the Paralympic programme are not as rigorously followed when it comes to female competitors. This tolerance is part of an attempt to actively recruit more women to the sport for the disabled. Thus men and women compete under different rules.

5 Mediated Paralympic culture

1 See the IPC website at www.paralympic.org for details of all the different roles and responsibilities the IPC undertakes.
2 This is a pseudonym for a weekly British track and field athletics publication.
3 In the past I have undertaken ethnographic research in the roles of Paralympic athlete and administrator. This experience made me a good fit as the first journalist from *Run, Throw and Jump* to cover the Paralympics onsite.
4 IPC, 'Pure Gold Medal for Paralympic Spirit' – Press Release, 19 September 2004; for more information on the prize see www.whangprize.org.

6 The imperfect body and sport

1 I use this term very loosely. My interest in sport for individuals with cerebral palsy was sparked by the fact that if I trained in a diligent manner, international travel would be my reward. In mainstream sport, such a goal was unattainable.
2 This is a term used to designate the leader of the delegation from a nation at an international sporting event.

7 Technology and the Paralympic Games

1 Club is an event for class F32/F51 athletes who either have very involved and severe cerebral palsy (F32) or a very high lesion on their spinal cord (F51), and as a result throwing a javelin is impractical and dangerous. The best athlete in this event is Stephen Miller from Great Britain. At the time of writing he was World Record Holder and Paralympic and World Champion in this event. The front cover of this monograph bears his image.
2 A push rim exists on the back wheels of most wheelchairs to allow for self-propulsion. On contemporary racing chairs these are much smaller than the back wheel, and as such the athletes' arms are able to work like pistons – pounding the rims at an angle that creates the most backward force to move the chair forward as quickly as possible.
3 www.ossur.com viewed 27 March 2007.
4 www.iaaf.org/news/Kind=512/newsId=38127.html viewed 27 March 2007.
5 http://www.cdpf.org.cn/ viewed 26 April 2007.

Bibliography

Allan, S. (1999) *News Culture*. Buckingham: Open University Press.

Albrecht, G. L. and Bury, M. (2001) 'The Political Economy of the Disability Market-place', in Albrecht, G. L., Seelman, K. D. and Bury, M. (eds) *Handbook of Disability Studies*. London: Sage, pp. 585–609.

Amit, V. (2000) 'Introduction: constructing the field', in Amit, V. (ed.) *Constructing the Field: Ethnographic Fieldwork in the Contemporary World*. London: Routledge, pp. 1–18.

—— (2002) 'Reconceptualizing Community', in Amit, V. (ed.) *Realizing Community: Concepts, Social Relationships and Sentiments*. London: Routledge.

Anderson, B. (1983) *Imagined Communities*. London: Verso.

Anderson, J. (2003) 'Turned into taxpayers: paraplegia, rehabilitation and sport at Stoke Mandeville, 1944–56', *Journal of Contemporary History*, 38(3), 461–475.

Andrews, D. L. (1993) 'Desperately seeking Michel: Foucault's genealogy, the body, and critical sport sociology', *Sociology of Sport Journal*, 10, 148–167.

APC Asian Paralympic Committee website (www. asianparalympic.org).

Appadurai, A. (1991) 'Global Ethnoscapes: Notes and Queries for a Transnational Anthropology', in Fox, R. G. (ed.) *Interventions: Anthropologies of the Present*. Santa Fe: School of American Research, pp. 191–210.

Armstrong, G. (1998) *Football Hooligans: Knowing the Score*. Oxford: Berg.

Armstrong, G. and Giulianotti, R. (eds) (1997) *Entering the Field: New Perspectives on World Football*. Oxford: Berg.

Atkinson, M. and Wilson, B. (2002) 'Bodies, Subcultures and Sport', in Maguire, J and Young, K. (eds) *Theory, Sport and Society*. Oxford: Elsevier, pp. 375–395.

Balding, C. (2004) 'Paralympics: Games I'll Never Forget', *The Observer*, 3 October.

—— (2005) 'Disabled Star Runs into Speed Trap', *The Observer*, 15 May.

Bale, J. (2004) *Running Culture: Racing in Time and Space*. London: Routledge.

Bannister, R. (1955) *First Four Minutes*. London: Putnam.

—— (1977) 'Review: Textbook of Sport for the Disabled', *Proceedings of the Royal Society of Medicine*, 70, 64.

Barnes, C. (1991) *Disabled People in Britain and Discrimination*. London: Hurst.

—— (1992) 'Qualitative research: valuable or irrelevant?', *Disability, Handicap and Society*, 7, 115–124.

Barnes, C. and Mercer, G. (1997) *Doing Disability Research*. Leeds: The Disability Press.

—— (2003) *Disability*. Oxford: Polity Press.

BBC (1994) 'Disability for dollars'. *On the Line*. London: BBC.

Becker, H. S. (1958) 'Problems of inference and proof in participant observation', *American Sociological Review*, 23(6), 652–660.

Berger, R. J. (2004) 'Pushing forward: disability, basketball, and me', *Qualitative Inquiry*, 10, 794–810.

Bernard, H. R. (1995) *Research Methods in Anthropology: qualitative and quantitative approaches*, 2nd edn. London: Alta Mira Press.

Blackshaw, T. and Crabbe, T. (2005) *New Perspectives on Sport and 'Deviance': Consumption, Performativity, and Social Control*. London: Routledge.

Blake, A. (1996) *The Body Language: The Meaning of Modern Sport*. London: Lawrence and Wishart.

Blanchard, K. (1995) *The Anthropology of Sport: An Introduction*, revised edn. London: Bergin and Garvey.

Borsay, A. (1998) 'Returning patients to the community: disability, medicine and economic rationality before the Industrial Revolution', *Disability & Society*, 13(5), 645–663.

—— (2004) *Disability and Social Policy in Britain Since 1750: A History of Exclusion*. London: Palgrave Macmillan.

Bossion, A. (1978) 'Sport and the young physically handicapped person', *Olympic Review*, 134, 708–716.

Botvin-Madorsky, J. G. (1986) 'Wheelchair sports medicine', *Western Journal of Medicine*, 144(6), 737–738.

Bourdieu, P. (1977) *Outline of a Theory of Practice*, Cambridge: Cambridge University Press.

—— (1984) *Distinction: A Social Critique of the Judgement of Taste*. London: Routledge.

—— (1988) 'Program for the sociology of sport', in Kang, S., MaAloon J. and DaMatta, R. (eds) *The Olympics and Cultural Exchange. Hanyang Ethnology Monograph No. 1*. Hanyang: Hanyang University Press.

—— (1990a) *The Logic of Practice*. Cambridge: Polity Press.

—— (1990b) *In Other Words: Essays Towards a Reflective Sociology*. London: Polity Press.

—— (1992) *The Logic of Practice*. Cambridge: Polity Press.

—— (1993) *Sociology in Question*. London: Sage.

Bourdieu, P. and Wacquant, L. (1992) *An Invitation to Reflective Sociology* Chicago: University of Chicago Press.

Bowen, J. (2002) 'The Americans with a Disabilities Act and its application to sport', *Journal of the Philosophy of Sport*, 29, 66–74.

Brooks, M. B. (1956) 'Prostheses for child amputees', *California Medicine*, 85, 293–298.

Brownell, S. (1995) *Training the Body for China: Sport in the Moral Order of the People's Republic*. London: University of Chicago Press.

Buckland, S. (2004) 'Kenny gears up for triple triumph', *Sunday Times*, 26 September.

Burgess, R. (1984) *In the Field: An Introduction to Field Research*. London: George Allen and Unwin.

Burnett, M. (2005) 'Olympic dreams of a blade runner', BBC online, 5 May (available at http://news.bbc.co.uk/sport1/hi/other_sports/disability_sport/4487443.stm) (viewed 27 March 2007).

Camilleri, J. M. (1999) 'Disability: a personal odyssey', *Disability and Society*, 14(6), 845–853.

Campbell, J. and Oliver, M. (1996) *Disability Politics: Understanding our Past, Changing our Future*. London: Routledge.

Cashman, R. (2006) *The Bitter Sweet Awakening: the Legacy of the Sydney 2000 Olympic Games*. Sydney: Walla Walla Press.

Chagnon, N. (1983) *Yanomamo: The Fierce People*. London: Thompson Learning.

Chaloner, E. J., Flora, H. S. and Ham, R. J. (2001) 'Amputations at the London Hospital 1852–1857', *Journal of the Royal Society of Medicine*, 94, 409–412.

Charles, J. M. (1995) Technology and the body of knowledge', *Quest*, 50, 379–388.

Charlton, J. (1998) *Nothing About Us Without Us: Disability, Oppression, and Empowerment*. London: University of California Press.

Chick, G. (1998) 'Leisure and culture: issues for an anthropology of leisure', *Leisure Sciences*, 20, 111–133.

Christie, J. (2004) '"Spirit in Motion": Paralympians Rise', *Globe and Mail*, 11 December.

Clement, J.-P. (1995) 'Contributions of the Sociology of Pierre Bourdieu to the Sociology of Sport', *Sociology of Sport Journal*, 12, 147–157.

Clifford, J. (1986) 'Introduction: Partial Truths', in Clifford, J. and Marcus, G. (eds) *Writing Culture: The Poetics and Politics of Ethnography*. Berkeley: University of California Press, pp. 1–26.

Clifford, J. and Marcus, G. (eds) (1986) *Writing Culture: The Poetics and Politics of Ethnography*. Berkeley: University of California Press.

Coffey, A. (1999) *The Ethnographic Self: Fieldwork and the Representation of Identity*. London: Sage.

Cole, B. A. (2005) 'Good faith and effort? Perspectives on educational inclusion', *Disability & Society*, 20, 331–344.

Cole, C. (1999) 'Faster, higher poorer', *National Post*, 28 August.

Cole, C. L., Giardina, M. D. and Andrews, D. L. (2004) 'Michel Foucault: Studies of Power and Sport', in Giulianotti, R. (ed.) *Sport and Modern Social Theorists*. Basingstoke: Palgrave MacMillan.

CP-ISRA (2001) *Classification and Sports Rule Manual*, 8th edn. CP-ISRA.

Crossley, N. (2001) *The Social Body: Habit, Identify and Desire*. London: Sage.

Csordas, T. (ed.) (1990) *Embodiment and Experience: the existential ground of culture and self*. Cambridge: Cambridge University Press.

—— (2002) *Body/Meaning/Healing*. New York: Palgrave Macmillan.

Cumberbatch, G. and Negrine, R. (1992) *Images of Disability on Television*. London: Routledge.

Daly, D. J. and Vanlandewijck, Y. (1999) 'Some criteria for evaluating the "fairness" of swimming classification', *Adapted Physical Activity Quarterly*, 16(3), pp. 271–289.

Davies, C. A. (1997) *Reflexive Ethnography: A Guide to Researching Selves and Others*. London: Routledge.

Davies, G. (2004) 'Canadian fails drug test', *Daily Telegraph*, 18 September.

Davis, L. J. (1995) *Enforcing Normalcy: Disability, Deafness and the Body*. London: Verso.

Davis, R. and Cooper, R. (1999) 'Technology for disabilities', *British Medical Journal*, 319, 1–4.

de Coubertin, P. (1956 [1935]) 'The fundamentals of the philosophy of the modern Olympics', *Bulletin de Comité International Olympique*, 56, 52–54.

de Garis, L. (1999) 'Experiments in pro wrestling: toward a performative and sensuous sport ethnography', *Sociology of Sport Journal*, 16, 65–74.

DePauw, K. (1997) 'The (In)Visibility of DisAbility: Cultural contexts and "sporting bodies",' *Quest*, 49, 416–430.

DePauw, K. and Gavron, S. (1995) *Disability and Sport*. Leeds: Human Kinetics.

—— (2005) *Disability Sport*, 2nd edn. Leeds: Human Kinetics Press.

DesGroseillers, J.-P., Desjardins, J.-P., Germain, J.-P. and Krol, A. L. (1978) 'Dermatologic problems in amputees', *Canadian Medical Association Journal*, 118, 535–537.

Dijkers, M. (1999) 'Community integration: conceptual issues and measurement approaches in rehabilitation research', *Journal of Rehabilitation Outcome Measurements*, 3(1), 39–49.

Doll-Tepper, G. (1999) 'Disability Sport', in Riordan, J. and Krüger, A. (eds) *The International Politics of Sport in the Twentieth Century*. London: E & FN Spon.

Douglas, M. (1966) *Purity and Danger*. London: Routledge.

Driedger, D. (1989) *Last Civil Rights Movement*. London: C. Hurst & Co.

Dummer, G. M. (1999) 'Classification of swimmers with physical disability', *Adapted Physical Activity Quarterly*, 16(3), 216–218.

Dyck, N. (2000) 'Introduction', in Dyck, N. (ed.) *Games, Sports and Cultures*. Oxford: Berg, pp. 1–9.

Edgerton, R. (1976) *Deviance: A Cross Cultural Perspective*. London: Benjamin and Cummings.

EPC (1999) *Europe News*, No. 5. European Paralympic Committee (April–July).

—— (2001) *Doping Disables*. Bonn. European Paralympic Committee.

Firth, R. (1931) 'A dart match in Tikopia', *Oceania*, 1, 64–97.

Fitzgerald, M. (2006) 'On a mission: Sarah Reinertsen is breaking new ground in sport and life', *Triathlete Magazine*, March, 104–111.

Foley, D. (1990) *Learning Capitalist Culture*. Philadelphia: University of Pennsylvania Press.

Foucault, M. (1973) *The Birth of the Clinic: An Archeology of Medical Perception*. London: Vintage Books.

—— (1977) *Discipline and Punish: The Birth of the Prison*. London: Harmondsworth.

Frossard, L., O'Riordan, A. and Goodman, S. (2006) 'Applied biomechanics for evidence based training of Australian elite seated throwers', *International Council of Sport Science and Physical Education Perspective Series*, pp. 1–12 (available at http://eprints.qut.edu.au/archive/00002713, retrieved 10 January 2007).

Geertz, C. (1973) *The Interpretation of Cultures*. New York: Basic Books.

Gerschick, T. J. and Miller, A. S. (1995) 'Coming to terms: masculinity and physical disability', in Sabo, D. and Gordon, D. F. (eds) *Men's Health and Illness: Gender, Power and the Body*. London: Sage, pp. 183–204.

Gilmour, G. (1963) *A Clean Pair of Heels: The Murray Halberg story*. Auckland: A.H. & A.W. Reed.

Giulianotti, R and Armstrong, G. 'Introduction: reclaiming the game – an introduction to the anthropology of football', in Armstrong, G. and Giulianotti, R. (eds) *Entering the Field: New Perspectives on World Football*. Oxford: Berg, pp. 1–29.

Gleeson, B. J. (1997) 'A historical materialist view of disability studies', *Disability & Society*, 12(2), 179–202.

Goffman, E. (1963) *Stigma: Notes on the Management of Spoiled Identity*. London: Penguin.

Goggin, G. and Newell, C. (2000) 'Crippling Paralympics? Media, disability and Olympism', *Media International Australia*, 97, 71–83.

Goodman, S. (1986) *Spirit of Stoke Mandeville: The Story of Ludwig Guttmann*. London: Collins.

Green, M. and Houlihan, B. (2005) *Elite Sport and Development: Policy Learning and Political Priorities*. London: Routledge.

Gruneau, R. (1991) 'Sport and "esprit de corps": notes on power, culture and the body', in Landry, F., Yerles, M. and Landry, M. (eds) *Sport: The Third Millennium*. Sainte-Foy, Quebec: Presses de l' Université Laval, pp. 169–186.

—— (1999 [1983]) *Class, Sport and Social Development*, 2nd edn. Leeds: Human Kinetics Press.

Guttmann, L. (1976) *Textbook of Sport for the Disabled*. Aylesbury: HM & M.

—— (1977a) 'The value of sport for the severely physically handicapped', *Olympic Review*, 111, 16–20, 45.

—— (1977b) 'Development of sport for the spinal paralysed', *Olympic Review*, 112, 110–113.

Hahn, H. (1984) 'Sports and the political movement of disabled persons: examining nondisabled values', *Arena Review*, 8, 1–15.

Hammersley, M. and Atkinson, P. (1989) *Ethnography: Principles in Practice*. London: Routledge.

—— (1995) *Ethnography: Principles and Practice*, 2nd edn. London: Routledge.

Haraway, D. J. (1991) *Simians, Cyborgs, and Women: The Reinvention of Nature*. London: Free Association Books.

Hargreaves, J. (2000) *Sporting Heroines*. London: Routledge.

Henderson, H. (2004) 'Golden opportunities: Paralympics is about empowering people through sport', *Toronto Star*, 11 September.

Hind, R. (2000) 'Sense and sensibilities: delicate balance of reporting the Paralympics', *Sydney Morning Herald*, 14 October.

Hoberman, John (1995) 'Toward a theory of Olympic internationalism', *Journal of Sports History*, 22(1), 1–37.

Hoberman, J. (1992) *Mortal Engineer: The Science of Performance and the Dehumanization of Sport*. Oxford: Maxwell Macmillan International.

Howe, P. D. (2001) 'An ethnography of pain and injury in professional rugby union: the case of Pontypridd RFC', *International Review of Sport Sociology*, 35(3), 289–303.

—— (2004a) *Sport, Pain and Professionalism: Ethnographies of Injury and Risk*. London: Routledge.

—— (2004b) Letter to the Sports Editor – 'As a four-time Paralympian', *The Observer*, 10 October.

—— (2006a) 'Habitus, Barriers and the [Ab]use of the Science of Interval Training in the 1950s', *Sporting History*, 26(2), 325–344.

—— (2006b) 'The role of injury in the Organisation of Paralympic Sport', in Loland, S., Skirstad, B. and Waddington, I. (eds) *Pain and Injury in Sport*. London: Routledge, pp. 211–226.

Howe, P. D. and Jones, C. (2006) 'Classification of disabled athletes: (dis)empowering the Paralympic practice community', *Sociology of Sport Journal*, 23, 29–46.

Howe, P. D. and Parker, A. (2005) 'Celebrating imperfection: sport, disability and celebrity culture', talk at 'Celebrity Culture: An Interdisciplinary Conference', Ayr, Scotland, UK, 12–14 September.

Hughes, B. (2000) 'Medicine and the aesthetic invalidation of disabled people', *Disability & Society*, 15(4), 555–568.

Hutchinson, N. (2006) 'Disabling beliefs? Impaired embodiment in the religious tradition of the West', *Body and Society*, 12(4), 1–23.

Ingham, A. and Donnelly, P. (1997) 'A sociology of North American sociology of sport: disunity in unity, 1965 to 1996', *Sociology of Sport Journal*, 14(4), 362–418.

IOC (2004) *Olympic Charter*. IOC.

IPC (2001) *The Paralympian: Newsletter of the International Paralympic Committee*, No. 3.

—— (2003a) *The Paralympian: Newsletter of the International Paralympic Committee*, No. 2.

—— (2003b) *The Paralympian: Newsletter of the International Paralympic Committee*, No. 3.

—— (2004) *The Paralympian: Official Newsletter of the International Paralympic Committee*, No. 1.

James, A., Hockey, J. and Dawson, A. (1997) 'Introduction: the road from Santa Fe', in James, A., Hockey, J. and Dawson, A. (eds) *After Writing Culture: Epistemology and Praxis in Contemporary Anthropology*. London: Routledge, pp. 1–15.

Jenks, C. (2005) *Subculture: The Fragmentation of the Social*. London: Sage.

Jennings, A. and Simson, V. (1992) *The Lords of the Rings: Power, Money and Drugs in the Modern Olympics*. London: Simon and Schuster.

Jones, C. and Howe, P. D. (2005) 'The conceptual boundaries of sport for the disabled: classification and athletic performance', *Journal of Philosophy of Sport*, 32, 133–146.

Kalbfuss, E. (2002) 'Petitclerc Rolls Home With Gold', *Gazette*, 5 August.

Kamenetz, H. L. (1969) 'A brief history of the wheelchair', *Journal of the History of Medicine*, April, 205–210.

Kelly, M. P. (2001) 'Disability and Community: A Sociological Approach', in Albrecht, G. L., Seelman, K. D. and Bury, M. (eds) *Handbook of Disability Studies*. London: Sage, pp. 396–411.

Kimayer, L. J. (2003) 'Reflections on Embodiment', in Wilce, J. M. (ed.) *Social Cultural Lives of Immune Systems*. London: Routledge, pp. 282–302.

Klein, A. (1991) *Sugarball: The American Game, the Dominican Dream*. New Haven: Yale University Press.

—— (1993) *Little Big Men: Bodybuilding Subculture and Gender Construction*. Albany: State University of New York.

Labanowich, S. (1988) 'A case for the integration of the disabled into the Olympic Games', *Adapted Physical Activity Quarterly*, 5, 264–272.

Laberge, S. and Kay, J. (2002) 'Pierre Bourdieu's Socialcultural Theory and Sporting Practice', in Maguire, J. and Young, K. (eds) *Theory, Sport and Society*. London: Elsevier Science, pp. 239–266.

Laberge, S. and Sankoff, D. (1988) 'Physical Activities, Body Habitus, and Lifestyles', in Harvey, J. and Cantelon, H. (eds) *Not Just a Game: Essays in Canadian Sport Sociology*. Ottawa: University of Ottawa Press.

Landry, F (1995) 'Paralympic Games and Social Integration' in de Moragas Spà, M. and Botella, M. (eds) *The Key of Success: The Social, Sporting, Economic and Communications Impact of Barcelona '92*. Bellaterra: Servei de Publicacions de la Universitat Autònoma de Barcelona, pp. 1–17.

Leder, D. (1990) *The Absent Body*. London: University of Chicago Press.

Lee, R. B. (1979) *The !Kung San: Men, Women, and Work, in a Foraging Society*. Cambridge, MA: Harvard University Press.

Legg, D., Emes, C., Stewart, D. and Steadward, R. (2004) 'Historical overview of the Paralympics, Special Olympics, and Dealympics', *Palaestra*, 20(1), 30–36.

Lesser, A. (1933) 'The Pawnee Ghost Dance Hand Game: A Study of Cultural Change', in *Columbia University Contribution to Anthropology*, No. 16. New York: Columbia University Press.

Lock, M. (1993) 'Cultivating the body: anthropology and epistemologies of bodily practice and knowledge', *Annual Review of Anthropology*, 22, 133–155.

Loland, S. (1995) Coubertin's Ideology of Olympism from the Perspective of the History of Ideas. *Olympika: the International Journal of Olympic Studies*, 4, 49–78.

—— (2002) *Fair Play in Sport: A Moral Norm System*. London: Routledge.

Lowe, M. (1999) *Inside the Sports Pages: Work Routines, Professional Ideologies and The Manufacture of Sports News*. Toronto: University of Toronto Press.

Lupton, D. (1995) *The Imperative of Health: Public Health and the Regulated Body*. London: Sage.

MacAloon, J. J (1981) *This Great Symbol: Pierre de Coubertin and the Origins of the Modern Olympic Games*. London: University of Chicago Press.

MacClancy, J. (1996) 'Sport, Identity and Ethnicity', in MacClancy, J. (ed.) *Sport, Identity and Ethnicity*. Oxford: Berg, pp. 1–20.

—— (ed.) (1996) *Sport, Identity and Ethnicity*. Oxford: Berg.

Marcus, G. and Fischer, M. (1986) *Anthropology as Cultural Critique: An Experimental Moment in Human Sciences*. Chicago: University of Chicago Press.

Markula, P. (2003) 'The technologies of the self: sport, feminism, and Foucault', *Sociology of Sport Journal*, 20, 87–107.

Markula, P. and Pringle, R. (2006) *Foucault, Sport and Exercise: Power, Knowledge and Transforming the Self*. London: Routledge.

Martin, J. J., Adams-Mushett, C. and Smith, K. L. (1995) 'Athletic identity and sport orientation of adolescent swimmers with disabilities', *Adapted Physical Activity Quarterly*, 12, 113–123.

Mason, F. (2002) 'Creating image and gaining control: the development of the Cooperation Agreements between the International Olympic Committee and the International Paralympic Committee', *VI International Symposium for Olympic Research*, pp. 113–122.

Mauss, M. (1990) *The Gift: The Form and Reason for Exchange in Archaic Societies*. London: W. W. Norton.

May, T. (1997) *Social Research: Issues, Methods and Process*, 2nd edn. Buckingham: Open University Press.

McCann, B. C. (1994) 'The Medical Disability – Specific Classification System in Sport', in Steadward, R. D., Nelson, E. R. and Wheeler, G. D. (eds) *Vista '93: The Outlook. Proceedings of the International Conference on High Performance Sport for Athletes with Disabilities*. Jasper, Alberta: Rick Hansen Centre, pp. 275–288.

McDonald, M. (2000) 'The XI Paralympic Games', *Olympic Review*, XXVI(34), 53–55.

Mennesson, C. (2000) '"Hard" women and "soft" women: the social construction of identity among female boxers', *International Review for Sociology of Sport*, 35(1), 21–33.

Merleau-Ponty, M. (1962) *Phenomenology of Perception*, London: Routledge and Kegan Paul.

—— (1965) *The Structure of Behaviour*. London: Methuen.

Miah, A. (2004) *Genetically Modified Athletes: Biomedical Ethics, Gene Doping and Sport*. London: Routledge.

Morgan, W. J. (1994a). *Leftist Theories of Sport: A Critique and Reconstruction*. Urbana: University of Illinois Press.

—— (1994b) 'Hegemony theory, social domination, and sport: the MacAloon and Hargreaves–Tomlinson debate revisited', *Sociology of Sport Journal*, 11, 309–329.

—— (2002) Social criticism as moral criticism: a Habermasian take on sport', *Journal of Sport and Social Issues*, 26, 281–299.

Morris, J. (1991) *Pride Against Prejudice: Transforming Attitudes to Disability*. London: Women's Press.

—— (1996) 'Introduction', in Morris, J. (ed.) *Encounter with Strangers: Feminism and Disability*. London: Women's Press.

Mosher, R. (1991) 'Special Olympics: Universal Games for the disabled', *Olympic Review*, 286, 380–383.

Mott, S. (2000) 'Impaired logic keeps heroes off the stage', *Daily Telegraph*, 11 December.

Murphy, R. F. (1987) *The Body Silent*. London: Dent.

Nadarajan, B. 'Sydney 2000 Paralympic Games: a coming of age', *Olympic Review*, XXVII(36), 5–8.

Nettleton, S. and Watson, J. (1998) 'The body in everyday life: an introduction', in Nettleton, S. and Watson, J. (eds) *The Body in Everyday Life*. London: Routledge, pp. 1–18.

Northway, R. (1997) 'Integration and inclusion: illusion or progress in services in services for disabled people', *Social Policy and Administration*, 31(2), 157–172.

Oliver, M. (1983) *Social Work with Disabled People*. London: Routledge.

—— (1990) *The Politics of Disablement*. London: Macmillan.

—— (1992) 'Changing the social relations of research production', *Disability, Handicap and Society*, 7, 101–114.

—— (1996) *Understanding Disability: From Theory to Practice*. London: Macmillan.

Oliver, M. and Barnes, C. (1998) *Social Policy and Disabled People: From Exclusion to Inclusion*. London: Longman.

O'Riordan, A. and Frossard, L. (2006) 'Seated shot put – what's it all about?', *Modern Athlete and Coach*, 44(2), 2–8.

Ortner, S. B. (2006) *Anthropology and Social Theory: Culture, Power and the Acting Subject*. London: Duke University Press.

Page, S. J., O'Connor, E. and Peterson, K. (2001) 'Leaving the disability ghetto: a qualitative study of factors underlying achievement motivation among athletes with disabilities', *Journal of Sport and Social Issues*, 25(1), 40–55.

Park, R. J. (1992) 'Athletes and Their Training in Britain and America, 1800–1914', in Berryman, J. W. and Park, R. J. (eds) *Sport and Exercise Science: Essays in the History of Sports Medicine*. Chicago: University of Illinois Press, pp. 57–107.

Park, S. J. (1987) 'Spirit of preparation', *Olympic Review*, 240, 500–501.

Parry, J. (2004) 'Olympism and its ethic', Paper presented at the 44th International Session of the International Olympic Academy, May/June.

Parsons, T. (1951) The Social System. London: Routledge and Kegan Paul.

Paterson, K. and Hughes, B. (1999) 'Disability studies and phenomenology: the carnal politics of everyday life', *Disability and Society*. 14(5), 597–610.

Peacock, J. L. (1986) *The Anthropological Lens: Harsh Light, Soft Focus*. Cambridge: Cambridge University Press.

Philips, R. (2005) 'Pistorius Masters Quick Step', *Telegraph*, 27 April.

Pingree, A. (1998) 'The development of the Paralympic Games: an interview with Dr. Robert Steadward', *Olympic Review*, XXVI(20), 58–60.

Pronger, B. (2002) *Body Fascism: Salvation in the Technology of Physical Fitness*. London: University of Toronto Press.

Pryor, M. (2004a) 'Lack of coverage undermines US bid', *Times*, 22 September.

—— (2004b) 'Athletes in front line of campaign to change perception', *Times*, 24 September.

—— (2004c) 'Sprinters have designs on rewriting records', *Times*, 23 September.

Quinn, M. (2006) 'Jeremy Bentham on Physical Disability: a problem for whom? Presented at 'Revisiting the Institution; Fresh Perspectives on the History of Physical Disability', Leeds University, 26 June.

Rail, G. and Harvey, J. (1995) 'Body at work: Michel Foucault and the sociology of sport', *Sociology of Sport Journal*, 12, 164–179.

Ravaud, J.-F. and Stiker, H.-J. (2001) 'Inclusion/Exclusion: An Analysis of Historical and Cultural Meaning', in Albrecht, G. L., Seelman, K. D. and Bury, M. (eds) *Handbook of Disability Studies*. London: Sage, pp. 490–512.

Reynolds-Whyte, S. and Ingstad, B. (1995) 'Disability and culture: an overview' in Ingstad, B. and Reynolds-Whyte, S. (eds) *Disability and Culture*. London: University of California Press.

Richter, K. J. (1994) 'Integrated Classification: An Analysis', in Steadward, R. D., Nelson, E. R. and Wheeler, G. D. (eds) *Vista '93: The Outlook. Proceedings of the International Conference on High Performance Sport for Athletes with Disabilities*. Jasper, Alberta: Rick Hansen Centre, pp. 255–259.

—— (1999) 'The Wheelchair Classification Debate'. Paper given at CP-ISRA STC, Ottawa, Canada, September.

Richter, K. J., Adams-Mushett, C., Ferrara, M. S. and McCann, B. C. (1992) 'Integrated swimming classification: a faulted system', *Adapted Physical Activity Quarterly*, 9, 5–13.

Riddell, S. and Watson, N. (2003a) (eds) *Disability, Culture and Identity*. Harlow: Pearson Education.

—— (2003b) 'Disability, Culture and Identity: Introduction', in Riddell, S. and Watson, N. (eds) *Disability, Culture and Identity*. Harlow: Pearson Education, pp. 1–18.

Robinson, L. (2000) 'Meet the real Olympians', *Globe and Mail*, 24 October.

Rossi, L. F. A (1974) 'Rehabilitation following below-knee amputation', *Proceedings of the Royal Society of Medicine*, 67, 37–38.

Rowe, D. (1999) *Sport, Culture and the Media*. Buckingham: Open University Press.

Sands, R. (1999a) 'Anthropology and sport', in Sands, R. (ed.) *Anthropology, Sport and Culture*. London: Bergin and Garve, pp. 3–14.

—— (ed.) (1999b) *Anthropology, Sport and Culture*. London: Bergin and Garvey.

—— (1999c) *Sport and Culture: At Play in the Fields of Anthropology*. Needham Heights: Simon and Schuster.

—— (2002) *Sport Ethnography*. Leeds: Human Kinetics.

Schantz, O. J. and Gilbert, K. (2001) 'An ideal misconstrued: newspaper coverage of the Atlanta Paralympic Games in France and Germany', *Sociology of Sport*, 18(1), 69–94.

Schell, L. A. and Duncan, M. C. (1999) 'A content analysis of CBS's coverage of the 1996 Paralympic Games', *Adapted Physical Activity Quarterly*, 16, 27–47.

Schell, L. A. and Rodriguez, S. (2001) 'Subverting bodies/ambivalent representations: media analysis of Paralympian, Hope Lewellen', *Sociology of Sport*, 18(1), 127–135.

Scheper-Hughes, N. and Lock, M. (1987) 'The mindful body: a prolegomenon to future work in medical anthropology', *Medical Anthropology Quarterly*, 1(1), 6–41.

Scruton, J. (1998) *Stoke Mandeville: Road to the Paralympics*. Aylesbury: The Peterhouse Press.

Seymour, W. (1998) *Remaking the Body: Rehabilitation and Change*. London: Routledge.

Shakespeare, T. and Watson, N. (1997) 'Defending the Social Model', *Disability and Society*, 12(2), 293–300.

—— (2002) 'The Social Model of Disability: an outdated ideology?' *Research in Social Science and Disability*, 2, 9–28.

Shephard, R. J. (1999) 'Postmodernism and adapted physical activity: a new gnostic heresy?', *Adapted Physical Activity Quarterly*, 16, 331–343.

Sherrill, C. (1990) 'Psychosocial status of disabled athletes', in Reid, G. (ed.) *Problems of Motor Control*. Amsterdam: North Holland, pp. 339–364.

—— (1999) 'Disability sport and classification theory: a new era'. *Adapted Physical Activity Quarterly*, 16, 206–215.

Sherrill, C. and Williams, T. (1996) 'Disability and sport: psychosocial perspectives on inclusion, integration and participation', *Sport Science Review*, 5(1), 42–64.

Shilling, C. (1993) *The Body and Social Theory*. London: Sage.

—— (2003) *The Body and Social Theory*, 2nd edn. London: Sage.

—— (2005) *The Body in Culture, Technology and Society*. London: Sage.

Shogan, D. (1998) 'The social construction of disability: the impact of statistics and technology', *Adapted Physical Activity Quarterly*, 15, 269–277.

—— (1999) *High-Performance Athletes: Discipline, Diversity, and Ethics*. Toronto: University of Toronto Press.

Simon, R. L. (1991) *Fair Play: Sports, Values, and Society*. Boulder: Westview Press.

Smart, B. (2005) *Modern Sport and the Cultural Economy of Sporting Celebrity*. London: Sage.

Smith, A. and Thomas, N. (2005) 'The "inclusion" of elite athletes with disabilities in the 2002 Manchester Commonwealth Games: an exploratory analysis of British newspaper coverage', *Sport, Education and Society*, 10, 49–67.

Smith, G. (1999) *Confronting the Present: Towards A Politically Engaged Anthropology*. Oxford: Berg.

Smith-Maguire, J. (2002) 'Michel Foucault: Sport, Power, Technologies and Governmentality', in Maguire, J. and Young, K. (eds) *Theory, Sport and Society*. London: Elsevier Science, pp. 293–314.

Sørensen, M. and Kahrs, N. (2006) 'Integration of disability sport in the Norwegian sport organizations: lessons learned', *Adapted Physical Activity Quarterly*, 23, 184–203.

Sparkes, A. C. (2002) *Telling Tales in Sport and Physical Activity: A Qualitative Journey*. Leeds: Human Kinetics.

Steadward, R. D. (1996) 'Integration and sport in the Paralympic Movement', *Sport Science Review*, 5(1), 26–41.

—— (2000) 'The Paralympic Movement: a championship future', *Proceedings of the 30th Session of the International Olympic Academy*. Lausanne: IOC.

Stone, E. (2001) 'Disability, sport, and the body in China', *Sociology of Sport Journal*, 18(1), 51–68.

Stone, S. D. (1995) 'The myth of bodily perfection', *Disability and Society*, 10(4), 413–424.

Sugden, J. (1996) *Boxing and Society: An International Analysis*. Manchester: University of Manchester Press.

—— (2005) 'Is investigative sociology just investigative journalism?', in McNamee, M. (ed.) *Philosophy and the Sciences of Exercise, Health and Sport*. London: Routledge.

Sugden, J. and Tomlinson, A. (1999) 'Digging the dirt and staying clean: retrieving the investigative tradition for a critical sociology of sport', *International Review for the Sociology of Sport*, 34(4), 385–397.

Taussig, M. (1980) *The Devil and Commodity Fetishism in South America*. London: University of North Carolina Press.

Thomas, C. (1999) *Female Forms: Experiencing and Understanding Disability*. Buckingham: Open University Press.

Thomas, N. and Smith, A. (2003) 'Preoccupied with able-bodiedness? An analysis of the British media coverage of the 2000 Paralympic Games', *Adapted Physical Activity Quarterly*, 20, 166–181.

Thompson, E. P. (1963) *The Making of the English Working Class*. London: Pantheon.

Thornton, S. (1995) *Club Cultures: Music, Media and Subcultural Capital*. Cambridge: Polity Press.

Tisdall, E. K. M. (2003) 'A culture of participation?', in Riddell, S. and Watson, N. (eds) *Disability, Culture and Identity*. London: Pearson Prentice Hall.

Topliss, E. (1979) *Provision for the Disabled*, 2nd edn. Oxford: Blackwell.

Turner, B. S. (1992) *Regulated Bodies: Essays in Medical Sociology*. London: Routledge.

—— 1996 *The Body and Society*, 2nd edn. London: Sage.

—— (2001) 'Disability and the Sociology of the Body', in Albrecht, G. L., Seelman, K. D. and Bury, M. (eds) *Handbook of Disability Studies*. London: Sage, pp. 252–266.

Turner, V. (1967) *The Forest of Symbols*. Ithaca: Cornell University Press.

—— (1969) *The Ritual Process: Structure and Anti-structure*. Chicago: University of Chicago Press.

Tylor, E. B. (1896) 'On American lot games as evidence of Asiatic intercourse before the time of Columbus', *International Archives for Ethnographia*, 9(Suppl.), 55–67.

Tyne, A. (1992) 'Normalisation: From Theory to Practice', in Brown, H. and Smith, H. (eds) *Normalisation: A Reader for the Nineties*. London: Routledge.

Tweedy, S. M. (2002) 'Taxonomic theory and the ICF: disability athletics classification', *Adapted Physical Activity Quarterly*, 19, 220–237.

UPIAS (1976) *Fundamental Principles of Disability*. London: Union of the Physically Impaired Against Segregation.

van de Ven, L., Post, M., de Witte, L. and van den Heuvel, W. (2005) 'It takes two to tango: the integration of people with disabilities into society', *Disability & Society*, 20(3), 311–329.

Vanlandewijck, Y. C. and Chappel, R. J. (1996) 'Integration and classification issues in competitive sports for athletes with disabilities', *Sport Science Review*, 5(1), 65–88.

Verbrugge, L. M. and Jette, A. M. (1994) 'The disablement process', *Social Science and Medicine*, 38(1), 1–14.

Wacquant, L. J. D. (1995) 'Pugs at work: body capital and bodily labour among professional boxers', *Body and Society*, 1(1), 65–93.

—— (2004) *Body and Soul: Notebooks of an Apprentice Boxer*. Oxford: Oxford University Press.

Ward, N. (1999) 'Foxing the nation: the economic (in)significance of hunting with hounds in Britain', *Journal of Rural Studies*, 15, 389–403.

Webling, D. D'A. and Fahrer, M. (1986) 'Early bent knee prostheses: ancestors of K9', *British Medical Journal*, 293, 1636–1637.

Wernick, A. (1991) *Promotional Culture: Advertising, Ideology and Symbolic Expression*. London: Sage.

West, P. (1985) 'Becoming Disabled: Perspectives on the Labelling Approach', in Gerhardt, U. E. and Wadworth, M. (eds) *Stress and Stigma*. London: Macmillan, pp. 104–128.

Whannel, G. (1992) *Fields of Vision: Television Sport and Cultural Transformation*. London: Routledge.

Wheaton, B. (1997) 'Covert Ethnography and the Ethics of Research: Studying Sport Subcultures', in Tomlinson, A. and Fleming, S. (eds) *Ethics, Sport and Leisure: Crises and Critiques*. Aachen: Meyer and Meyer, pp. 163–171.

—— (2000) 'Just do it: consumption, commitment, and identity in windsurfing subculture', *Sociology of Sport Journal*, 17(3), 254–274.

Wheaton, B. and Tomlinson, A. (1998) 'The changing gender order in sport? The case of windsurfing subcultures', *Journal of Sport and Social Issues*, 22(3), 252–274.

White, P. G., Young, K. and McTeer, W. G. (1995) 'Sport, Masculinity and the Injured

Body', in Sabo, D. and Gordon, F. (eds) *Men's Health and Illness: Gender, Power, and the Body*. London: Sage.

Williams, G. and Busby, H. (2000) 'The politics of "disabled" bodies', in Williams, S. J., Gabe, J. and Calnan, M. (eds) *Health, Medicine and Society: Key Theories, Future Agendas*. London: Routledge, pp. 169–185.

Williams, R. (1977) *Marxism and Literature*. Oxford: Blackwell.

Williams, T. (1994a) 'Disability sport socialisation and identity construction', *Adapted Physical Activity Quarterly*, 11, 14–31.

—— (1994b) 'Sociological perspectives on sport and disability: structural-functionalism', *Physical Education Review*, 17(1), 14–24.

Wolff, E. A., Torres, C. and Hums, M. A. (2007) 'Olympism and the Olympic athlete with a disability', in Schantz, O. and Gilbert, K. (eds) *The Paralympics: Elite Sport or Freak Show?* New York: Meyer & Meyer.

Wong, J. (2004) 'Nation Builder 2004: Chantel Petitclerc', *Globe and Mail*, 11 December.

Woods, B. and Watson, N. (2004) 'The social and technical history of wheelchairs', *International Journal of Therapy and Rehabilitation*, 11(9), 407–410.

Wu, S. K. and Williams, T. (1999) 'Paralympic swimming performance, impairment, and the functional classification system', *Adapted Physical Activity Quarterly*, 16(3), 251–270.

Wu, S. K., Williams, T. and Sherrill, C. (2000) 'Classifiers as agents of social control in disability swimming', *Adaptive Physical Activity Quarterly*, 17, 421–436.

Yilla, A. B. (2000) 'Enhancing Wheelchair Sport Performance', in Winnock, J. (ed.) *Adapted Physical Education and Sport*, 3rd edn. Leeds: Human Kinetics, pp. 419–431.

—— (2004) 'Anatomy of the sports wheelchair', *Athletic Therapy Today*, May, 33–35.

Zola, I. K. (1989) 'Towards the necessary universalizing of disability policy', *The Millbank Memorial Fund Quarterly*, 67(Suppl.), 401–428.

Index